Kundalini Awakening
for
Personal Mastery

Robert Morgen

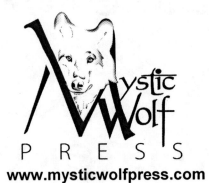

www.mysticwolfpress.com

ISBN 13: 978-0-9773801-0-7
ISBN 10: 0-9773801-0-6

Library of Congress Control Number: 2005935320

First Printing October 2005

Author photo by Anya Yankelevich

Printed in the USA

The Journey to Personal Mastery

We all dream of becoming more than we are at this moment and most of us feel intuitively that we have abilities and powers that we haven't unlocked yet.

Awakening the Kundalini is the beginning of a life changing journey that reveals our hidden powers and abilities, unlocks the mystery of life and helps us become the people we were born to be.

If you have the courage and the patience to really get to know yourself and unlock your hidden potential then this book can get you started on the right path.

Disclaimer

Awakening the Kundalini can cause extreme changes in ones personality and physical, mental and emotional health. Done properly these changes are positive and can result in the seeker developing remarkable abilities as well as deeper connections to the universe and their own spirituality.

Done improperly these changes can result in paranoia, schizophrenia and depression.

The exercises and meditations in this book were created to help awaken the Kundalini in a positive, healthy manner. There's nothing in this book that the author hasn't personally experienced.

Once you step onto this path there's literally no going back as the exercises and meditations in this book can awaken new abilities and personality changes in the seeker. YOU as the seeker have complete and sole responsibility for anything that happens beyond this point.

Other books and products
by Robert Morgen

Easy Meditation for Martial Artists

Basic Meditation for Druids (Coming in 2007)

Your Perfect Life (Coming in 2007)

Meditation CD's

Easy Introduction to Meditation

Advanced Meditation Exercises

Timed Meditations

Opening the Chakras

Easy Meditation CD Set (includes all 4 CD's)

Kundalini Awakening with Robert Morgen
Podcast

Robert Morgen produces a FREE Podcast in which you may download many of the exercises from this book as *guided meditations.*

You may access this Podcast at the Mystic Wolf Press website at: www.mysticwolfpress.com

About the Author

Robert Morgen is a Reiki Master who holds a Black Belt in Hoshinjutsu, a Brown Belt in Combat Hapkido and is the founder of the Mystic Village Online Community at *www.mysticvillage.org*

He's also the founder and moderator of the Kundalini Awakening Discussion Group at:
www.care2.com/c2c/group/Kundalini

He writes a regular column on subtle (or internal) energy for *Fight Times Magazine* and a column on Kundalini Awakening at *Kundalini Awakening Online* Magazine. He's the author of 3 books and 4 CDs on meditation and energy work.

He's a member of the Order of Bards, Ovates and Druids as well as the International Bujinkan Dojo Association, Canemasters International and the International Combat Hapkido Federation.

He travels and teaches as much as possible and you can learn more about his books, Kundalini and Martial Arts Seminars and FREE newsletter and events at his website.

"Robert Morgen's Easy Meditation CD Set" is also available at Amazon.com, retail outlets around the country and directly from the publisher at:

www.mysticwolfpress.com

Contents

Dedication

For Anya, for standing by me when it didn't make any sense. For Jake for being so much fun.

For my sister Karen, for all the years of wondering what was wrong with me. ☺
For Andy for being so cool.

For Jeff, Lynda, Jan, Doug, Brian, Jen and Pete because good friends are nice to have and when you can list them all that easily then you should.

For Glenn Morris for making things make sense, even when it hurt (a lot ☺).

ॐ

Introduction:

Surrender

I was lying paralyzed on a table in the emergency room in a Ft. Lauderdale hospital, wondering what to do next.

It started as a fun day at the beach, a day-after-Thanksgiving picnic with my sister, her boyfriend and my nephew. I remember the sense of joy and happiness as I ran towards the water, watching the blue of the Atlantic turn into white foam as the waves crashed in towards the beach.

I remember the feel of the water as I dove into it, and the shock of my forehead hitting the bottom as my entire body went completely numb. I knew instantly that I'd dove in too shallowly, a stupid, careless mistake. I didn't waste too much time thinking about that though, as solving my predicament required a certain amount of focus. Rather than fight against the paralysis, I relaxed completely, thankful for my years of training as a scuba diver. I held my breath and floated back up to the surface, thinking to myself "OK this is good, I've pinched a nerve or something and now I'm lying facedown in the Atlantic Ocean, holding my breath. I guess things could be worse."

Then a wave hit and rolled me slightly face up, just for a second. I quickly took another breath, the wave released me and I fell back face-down again. I don't know how many times this cycle was repeated. I only knew that all I could do was lie there and wait to see when, or if, that next breath would come. After an eternity that only turned out to be a minute or two, my sister's boyfriend and the lifeguard, a 3rd semester paramedic student, were able to get to me. The lifeguard got me turned over and, suspecting a spinal injury, immediately took steps to stabilize my head and spine until the ambulance could get there.

In the meantime the paralysis hadn't shown any signs of abating. I could breathe and feel my heart beating, but nothing else, and very recent experience had shown me how fragile reliance on the breath could be. I remember feeling very calm, even though I was literally scared for my life. I was constantly aware of the motion of the ambulance, and knew from my time as a Navy Hospital Corpsman how fragile spinal wounds could be. At any moment I expected that last remnant of my spinal cord to break and the signals from my brain to my heart and lungs to cease, and I knew there was absolutely nothing I could do about it. I remember very clearly the way the ambulance bounced as it crossed the railroad tracks and the moment when I decided that I couldn't be afraid anymore. I'd just have to accept the situation exactly as it was. I didn't have any choice.

I relaxed mentally and resolved that if I was going to die of stupidity then I least I wouldn't die scared out of my wits. By now I was in the ER and I was aware of the doctors giving orders and the nurses asking me questions. I remember the needles and catheters and canulas, but my mind wasn't focused on that.

At the time I was still conventionally religious (Methodist, I didn't know any better) and the only place I could turn was the Christian idea of God.

"Lord", I thought as I lay among the hustling medics, "I can't move anything but my eyelids and I don't know what's going to happen. I only know that I want to make the best out of whatever happens. If I'm supposed to die here, well, I can't do anything about that. I can't fight this physically and I accept that. I'm not gonna make any deathbed promises, I'm surrendering completely to whatever happens and I'll do what I can to make the best of it."

So I lay there and relaxed and waited for the clouds to part or for some sign while they prepped me for X-rays and got me stabilized. Nothing happened. We got back from the X-ray department and I lay there for a long time, beginning to get more relaxed and beginning to believe that I was going to live.

was also a Reiki Master, so he introduced me to Reiki, as well as Chi Kung.

Over the next decade I floundered around (or so I thought), working a wide variety of jobs and studying a strange variety of classes in school. I also spent a large amount of time out in the mountains or hiding out in the desert and just communing and doing various types of energy work.

A few years ago while living up in Glenwood Springs, CO, I was again drawn to get deeper into my energy work, and entered a period of intense yoga, Reiki, chi kung and meditation practice. One night while meditating I had a vision of a lotus flower, but the vision included the flower, the stem and the roots. The meaning was instantly obvious and I easily connected my energy. I felt a rush of energy up my spine and out through the top of my head.

Over the next few months I went through a period that I can only describe as a karmic clean-out. Any unresolved issue that I didn't deal with properly would keep popping up over and over until I dealt with it calmly and from my center. During a period when I was just being hired by UPS, I had my driver's license revoked twice, blew the engines on 3 vehicles and had a tortured series of bureaucratic battles. I had strange energy surges as my body re-wired itself. The resulting energy releases sent me to massage therapists and other Reiki practitioners to have them cleaned out. Some of this still happens, and probably always will.

I also went through a period of balancing my chakras, and I can look back at my life in various periods and see which chakra was dominant during that period.

After a few months I started trying to get away from it all. I stopped doing my yoga and meditation and entered a period that I can only describe as a mental hell. I later learned that, even at that time, I was balancing out my light and dark sides.

After a few months of this I finally realized that the best way to deal with all this was to *quit trying to deal with it and JUST ACCEPT IT.*

Once I began relaxing into myself and wasn't fighting the changes as much, I began to feel a deep connection to the other energy around me. Cities like Denver drove me nuts, and a casual drive through the mountains (my buddy Jeff called them 'medicine drives') would turn into an hours long meditation as I could feel the energy of all the trees and the world around me as I passed through.

At the time I was living in an old RV and just traveling around. It was still a time of healing and I carried around a damaged feeling that was gradually lessening as I became more relaxed. I went back to Albuquerque for the winter and, even though things were still hard, I was learning to feel better.

Then one day in February I suddenly realized that I was still working against myself. I made a silent affirmation that I would just relax, have fun and enjoy each moment and see where I was supposed to go next.

A couple of days later I got a message from Jeff that Dr. Glenn Morris (whom I'd finally had a chance to meet at a metaphysical fair the previous October) wanted me to come up to Denver for a weekend and assist with his booth at another metaphysical fair. So back I came to Denver, and a weekend of volunteer work turned into a temporary partnership in a nonprofit and work with several of Dr. Morris's Kundalini awakening seminars.

My training with Glenn Morris opened up a vast world of new experiences and showed me that so many parts of my life actually made sense, and opened the way for the healing and growth that I needed so badly.

Along the way I remembered that every time I had a problem or needed some direction I could just relax and affirm to go wherever I was supposed to.

The lesson for me was to have a little faith, and that having faith will work only if you commit to it. Have faith and be willing to go wherever you're needed and everything else will follow. Even now I continue to affirm that I'll go wherever I'm supposed to go and do whatever it is that I'm supposed to do, and so far I've ALWAYS had the guidance I needed within a couple of days.

Even now I learn and experience new things, and hopefully always will. Some of the lessons I've learned have been painfully hard, but worth it in the end. I hope the exercises and essays in this book will make your journey a little smoother than mine was in the beginning.

Part 1

Kundalini Basics

2   Personal Mastery

Chapter 1

What is Kundalini?

Kundalini is a Sanskrit word for a pool of energy that lies at the base of the spine. Dormant in most people, Kundalini energy can be awakened. It subsequently travels up the spine, activating the chakras and completing the body's energy circuits.

Kundalini can be awakened by a near-death experience, a mental, physical or emotional trauma, or by meditation and study. The completion of these energy circuits can bring out many different effects in the student/victim. Many people who experience a spontaneous awakening find themselves on new spiritual or life paths. Some people also have massive changes to their personalities as well as numerous benefits to their health. Some of the unlucky victims of the spontaneous awakenings can also experience epilepsy, depression and paranoia. It's my belief that many of the people we treat medically for these problems have, in fact, accessed this energy but are unfortunate enough to live in a world where its uses are relatively unknown and are for the most part unrecognized or misunderstood.

The seeker who purposefully awakens their Kundalini can discover increases in energy at the physical, mental, emotional and spiritual levels that frequently cause them to see the world and its inhabitants in a much different way than the ordinary person. Kundalini adepts can experience noticeable gains in psychic abilities, sensory perceptions and overall physical health, as well as a new spiritual outlook. All of these dramatic effects are caused by the realization and integration of the seeker's entire *self* into the greater consciousness of the universe. In short, the seeker can now actually feel his or her place in the interconnectedness of all things.

The Kundalini as a goal

One of the best ways to sabotage your practice is to set Kundalini Awakening as your *goal*. Awakening your Kundalini should be a side effect of a good practice, rather than the goal. It's important to be clear on this from the beginning.

When you have a good meditation practice, then you'll be automatically working towards awakening your Kundalini. You don't ever have to give the Kundalini another thought. It'll happen when you're ready for it and when you can handle the growth and the changes that it brings about. I've seen people who were completely focused on the Kundalini, to the extent that they would scan the Table of Contents of a book and only read the chapters directly concerned with the Kundalini.

The shortsightedness of this is the fact that the Kundalini is all about connecting ourselves to a limitless pool of all-encompassing energy and by limiting themselves this way they actually send out a message to the universe that they aren't really interested in the whole package, just these certain parts of it. The result is an extremely unbalanced person.

DON'T look at the Kundalini as the end-all, be-all. It's just another experience on the path. It's like crossing a small stream, now you're on the other side and ready to continue the journey. Just do your practice and learn to BE, and the Kundalini will take care of itself. When it does I'll bet you'll find the transition to be less life altering, and therefore easier.

6   Personal Mastery

Chapter 2

Kundalini History

Kundalini is from the Sanskrit word "Kundal" meaning 'coiled' which refers to the coil of energy resting at the base of the spine in the sacrum. The terms 'Serpent Power' and 'Serpent Energy' come from seeing this coiled energy as a snake.

Throughout history the serpent has been used as a symbol for Kundalini awakening. The Biblical story of Adam and Eve is viewed by many as an example of Kundalini Awakening. Adam and Eve are seen as the male/female energies and the "Serpent in the Garden" seen as the awakening of the human spirit to the realities that surround us. The Egyptians and the Greeks also used the serpent to represent knowledge.

The ancient symbol of the Caduceus used by our modern medical profession is seen to represent the 3 energy channels of the body. The Ida and Pingalla are represented by the twin serpents coiled around the staff, while the staff itself is seen as the Sushumna, or the middle channel through which the Kundalini ascends. Going back even further, about 4,000 years ago the Sumerian God Ningishita was represented by a single serpent coiled around a staff.

In Egypt the spinal cord was symbolized by the serpent and the cobra on the Pharaohs forehead represented the *divine fire* which had crawled serpent-like up the tree of life.

Another Biblical figure, Moses, also uses serpent energy in the liberation of his people from the Egyptians. History is filled with examples of the Kundalini, but most people simply don't recognize them. By the time you finish this book you'll be able to recognize the Kundalini in a huge variety of books, historical examples and even modern movies. It can be a lot of fun to see the clues that are hidden right out in the open. What makes them hidden is simply the fact that most people have no clue that the Kundalini exists or what it's about.

Chapter 3

Kundalini in Everyday Life

"To know the not-Self in one's nature is the pathway to knowledge of the Self."
N. Sri Ram, Thoughts for Aspirants

Making Changes

Kundalini awakening is about becoming the person we're meant to be. Awakening the Kundalini is a fairly simple process and to be honest it's not even all that hard to do. The real challenge with the Kundalini is in surrendering to it and going where it leads.

When you set out on the path to awaken your Kundalini you begin a growth process which by its very nature becomes a one way trip. As you study and grow and learn you'll go through incremental changes which will inevitably turn you into a different person. In this sense the Kundalini awakening becomes sort of a chicken/egg process i.e. "did you have massive personality changes because your Kundalini awakened or did your Kundalini awaken because you made massive personality changes?"

Kundalini awakening is a process of *becoming* an 'enlightened being'. No one just wakes up one day as an enlightened master; it's a process that they undertook over a long period of time that made extreme changes to the way they look at the world and the way they react to it on a moment to moment basis. The only way to *become* a master is to spend a lot of time BE-ing masterful in every moment.

Keeping a journal

The first time I read *Pathnotes of an American Ninja Master*, Dr. Glenn Morris mentions the fact that if you follow this path you're going to be making some extreme changes to your life and that you should keep a journal. Now, a decade and a half later, as I look back on all the things that have happened and the places I've been, I realize that as usual, he's exactly right. I didn't keep a journal however, so when I urge you to begin keeping one right now it's through my own bad example. Someday when you try to write a book to explain how you got to be the way you are (or at least the way you'll be then), you'll wish you had.

I bring this up because you'll see many instances in this book where I learned the hard way rather than just following the good advice of someone who's already been where I'm trying to go. Just something to think about.

Kundalini questions

This is from an email that someone sent me. You'll notice that I also used part of it later on in the book also. I include it here to illustrate that sometimes the Kundalini awakens spontaneously, which can be a real shock when the victim doesn't have the first clue what's happening to them.

Alex Wrote;

"What is the difference after the Kundalini awakens, and how do you know if it did?

About 25 years ago I was sitting alone by a creek in the morning, not formally meditating (which I've never done), just watching the water flow.

Suddenly there was an extremely intense ball of energy that formed at the base of my spine, buzzed there for a bit, then shot up my spine and 'exploded' in my head and 'out my eyes' and turned what I saw into a sort of mosaic made of the colors of what was there, but not the exact forms anymore.

A 2nd less intense one happened about 15 sec after the first. It scared me and I kind of blinked myself out of it.

Is that a Kundalini awakening, and if not, do you know what it was? If it was, how do you specifically use it?
Thanks,
Alex"
Hi Alex,

You've asked a great question that really hits at the heart of Kundalini awakening. Having said that, there's no short answer. You really weren't expecting a YES or a NO were you? :)

At its most basic level awakening the Kundalini completes the energy circuit between your 'potential energy' (dormant Kundalini) and your 'spiritual energy' (those are my terms and they merely serve to signify the differences in the energy. Other folks name them differently.) at your crown chakra. To paraphrase Glenn Morris "The Kundalini just connects your (genitals) to your brain."

Along the way it tends to begin the process of awakening and cleansing and balancing your chakras and cleaning out the rest of your body. Everyone experiences it differently because everyone *is* different at that level and we all get what we *need* individually. That's why some folks refer to the Kundalini (Shakti) as 'intelligent' energy.

So here's where it gets sticky. *Everyone* who's experienced a Kundalini awakening reports differently about it, and any external guidelines about what you *should* feel are merely that and can only be taken at face value, which is pretty close to nothing. :)

Some people experience very dramatic and extreme effects when their Kundalini awakens, and some hit it like a minor speed bump and keep right on going the way they were.

Some people end up on medication or in an asylum, while some give away all their possessions and pursue a spiritual path (which can also lead to asylums, medication and being nailed to the closest available tree). Others just continue on their pre-chosen path almost as if nothing happened.

There are a lot of human variables in the above experiences and outcomes, just like anything else. For some people the grand realizations are too much to deal with, or the siddhis (magics, extra-sensory perceptions that some people experience) may just be too much to handle. Others simply don't recognize what's happened to them, and you have to face it, we live in a society that doesn't accept this as part of the norm, so it becomes a curse rather than a cure.

Others pursue it as a stepping stone (rather than the destination) on the path to personal mastery. Some seek it as the precursor to Enlightenment and pursue it as if attaining it gives them some sort of bonus like reduced auto insurance rates.

Some of the Enlightenment seekers have actually managed to turn Kundalini awakening into an ego-driven fad, which I find to be extremely amusing.

Enlightenment only exists as a relative term. There's complete ignorance and lack of awareness on one end of the scale, and Enlightenment on the other. Neither exists independently, but rather as a moment to moment reaction to what's going on (going Om? Wisdom from the Land of Freudian

Typo's?) around us. Is true enlightenment simply recognizing the connections that we all have to one another and *really* treating others as we'd want to be treated, loving others as we should love ourselves?

Awakening the Kundalini or spending a decade in a cave on a mountain doesn't necessarily make one enlightened. Spending *every* moment actually *in* the moment and responding to the same divine spark in others that we also have within us possibly does.

One of the things that Kundalini awakening does for a lot of people is get them onto the path they came here (this lifetime) to pursue, hence the dramatic lifestyle changes. Others may always have been on the right path and didn't need the dramatic changes.

In my case the Kundalini was sort of like a hidden clue that I left myself before coming back to this life. Once I finally began to pay attention to what was happening (and being particularly dense it was quite a ride) then I was able to finally put a lifetime of strangely jumbled experiences into a real order that made sense and see where it all ties in together and what I'm supposed to do with it. That doesn't mean that I always (or even frequently) get it 'right', but at least I'm to the point where learning the lessons is easier and I can get it through my thick melon with a little less suffering (he said hopefully). :)

As to this question;
">What is the difference after the
> Kundalini awakens, and how do you know
if it did?"

The answer is completely up to you
and really can't be verified externally. It's all
about your own self-awareness and your un-
self-awareness. There are various signs that
you can go by which help, but unfortunately
it's not as simple as passing a test and
getting certified.

My first Kundalini awakening
happened while I was in the hospital during
a near-death experience, but I didn't
recognize that til over a decade later, in spite
of the dramatic things that I experienced. It
was only years later when I began to meet
others who had experienced it and learn
more about it that I realized what had
happened.

So the short answer that I can give you
is MAYBE. :)

As to "...how to specifically use it"? I
can tell you that *exactly*. :)

What you do to specifically use it is
relax and surrender to it and see where it
takes you. This requires a certain amount of
faith and a willingness to go where it leads,
which can obviously be pretty scary. A
positive attitude is an absolute necessity
here as the Kundalini will enhance and
magnify whatever you *are*, so spend your
time BE-ing something that should be
magnified.

As Glenn Morris once said during a seminar "The Kundalini magnifies you, so if you were an asshole before you awakened then afterwards you become wide and gaping".

I hope all that helps,

Robert :)

Creating your personal catalog of experiences

I was at a Reiki Share once and there was a very interesting young man there who was clearly experiencing some awakening energy. As we talked about his experiences he'd start to describe them and then stop, slightly embarrassed, and then say "Well, this may just be bullshit, but this is what I felt..."

After about the third or fourth time he did this I just stopped him and said "Look, if you experienced it then that makes it real. Nobody has the right to tell you that you didn't. There IS NO external validation for a lot of this stuff! It's *all* about learning to feel things and then *trust* your feelings."

Many of the exercises and drills in this book are about helping you to access and learn to use your internal energies. They're also about helping you to recognize what's going on in your world and to understand what's happening to you. *You* are the only person who can decide if what you're feeling is real and then categorize it properly. This is all about building up your own personal catalog of experiences.

One of the things that makes teaching *subtle energy* so difficult (and so easy for the charlatan, in some cases) is that the energies *are* subtle. In many cases it takes people a long time to really connect to the energy and understand that connection. I did the Microcosmic Orbit for over 2 *years* before I really felt the connection and began to figure it out. I can tell you what something feels like for me, but I can't tell you what it should feel like for you.

That's why I say over and over again to keep a positive attitude and play with this stuff. It's the only way to discover what it feels like.

Karma

We hear a lot about Karma. This is good karma, you have bad karma, etc. Most people are of the opinion that karma is the result of your last life coming back to bite you in the ass in this one. I only partially agree. I also think we make our own karma as we go and have to deal with it in this life.

Karma is simply the results of our actions. For example, if you frequently use anger as a tool then you have to expect to be put in positions where anger is necessary. You create that circle and then perpetuate it. In part it goes back to the Law of Reciprocity and in part it has to do with our subconscious. Some Kundalini teachers will tell you that the Kundalini breaks the wheel of karma. I agree but I don't think it works the way most people think.

When I say that the Kundalini breaks the wheel of karma then what I mean is that it forces you to examine yourself in such detail that you'll have to clean up your messes, even those that carried over from past lives. I don't see the Kundalini as some karmic 'get out of hell free' card. Rather it's like a huge mirror that doesn't lie to you and won't let you lie to yourself.

As you go through the period of cleansing and balancing your chakras you'll have the opportunity to look at yourself and your life very closely. My advice is to make the time to do this on your on and begin the process yourself rather than having it dumped on you all at once. It's all part of the self-awareness training that you'll be doing for the rest of your life.

As you develop the level of self-awareness that lets you be in constant control of your actions you'll be able to move your karma in positive directions. To use the earlier example of anger, by showing more compassion to angry people *you'll* be given more compassion on those occasions that you slip off the wagon and become angry yourself.

The Transition to Awakening

There are a lot of things you can do to make this entire process easier. You'll see these mentioned over and over throughout this book, primarily because they work. Kundalini Awakening doesn't have to be a huge, dramatic, life altering shock to your system. The following techniques can make it much easier.

Have Faith

Faith is an important component in Kundalini awakening because you have to surrender your egotistical sense of control and be willing to go where you're sent. You have to *believe* absolutely that you're doing the right thing. You can have faith in a limitless number of Gods both modern and ancient or you can make up your own. They're all just symbols of the eternal energy of creation and you can personify them to your hearts content, just as long as you truly have faith.

Personally I don't bother with any of the common deities. I think we as humans have such an amazingly small viewpoint that we wouldn't recognize a real god if we got into bed with it. It's like a couple of ants trying to discuss a human. For me it's enough to feel the "universal energy" of creation and just believe in that.

Of course to have faith you have to believe that the energy is intelligent and directed, otherwise why would it matter if you had faith in it or not? I do believe that, but that's as far as I've bothered to think about it, because beyond that it really doesn't matter. It's enough to accept it at a soul level and trust it. Whatever *it* is.

Keeping a Positive Attitude

"The Kundalini just magnifies whatever you are. If you were an asshole before the Kundalini then afterwards you become wide and gaping."
Dr. Glenn Morris
Author of *Pathnotes of an American Ninja Master*

As you begin to follow this path you're going to experience emotions, feelings and in some cases pain. Sometimes it'll only make sense years later when you look back on it and realize what was happening. In many cases awakening the Kundalini is like trying to put together a jigsaw puzzle without having any kind of picture to go by.

No matter what happens, or where you feel drawn to go, a positive attitude will make the whole thing easier. I try to look at *everything* as a test, and that works for my personality. Each individual moment I have choices that I can make. I can be enlightened or ignorant, loving or afraid, loud or quiet and it all depends on my willingness to listen to the inner voices that we all have. The *inner voices* (spirit guides?)(Yeah, I *know* it sounds crazy) are an amazing asset to keeping you on the right path and helping you become the person you came here to be.

That kind of insanity requires a positive attitude.

Developing your self-awareness

"Asking good questions is half of learning."
Muhammad
Essential Sufism

Kundalini awakening begins with the process of learning exactly who you are, with all your warts, wonders and blemishes. Once you've done that and become completely at ease with your self acceptance then you can promptly just forget all of it and disappear into the ether. Literally.

Your *self* is just like a blanket that you cover up with or a jacket that you put on. Spend some time becoming completely comfortable with it and you'll begin to see that you can put it on and take it off at will. It's just an external way to identify which *self* is yours. Once you can get beyond that and see that *you* don't really exist, then you can really start having fun with this stuff.

Developing your self-awareness is a multi-faceted exercise that encompasses all parts of your being. No matter how good you become at it there will always be new layers to uncover and new things to learn.

At the elementary levels of this book we'll look at your physical self, your mental self and your spiritual self and see how we can integrate them into your total being.

Yoga, martial arts and physical fitness

You don't have to be in excellent physical condition to awaken your Kundalini, but it helps. Your body is what you live in while you're here. I'm always amazed by the people who insist on having a nice house or a big, fancy car, yet ignore the one vehicle they can't live without.

I always advise people to get into a good yoga practice for several reasons.

1. Our bodies store memories, feelings and stresses within our muscles and organs. Yoga helps release those stresses in a relaxed, gradual manner, rather than all at once through a chakra-ic cleansing.

2. When you breathe properly during the yoga positions (asanas) then you're also massaging your internal organs as well as stretching your muscles. This provides an immediate health benefit as well as helping to release stored toxins and feelings.

3. Yoga lubricates and relaxes the spine, allows you to move more easily and freely and adds a much better quality of life. A relaxed healthy spine is also a better conduit for chi.

4. "Energy doesn't flow through tight muscles" (you'll hear that over and over again). The relaxing effects of a good yoga practice help prevent muscle tightness that can impede your energy flow.

Some forms of the martial arts such as Tai Chi, Chi Kung, Tai Jutsu and Hoshin Roshi Ryu help build remarkable energy awareness and strength. They also help you become more confident and comfortable in your surroundings. In my Hoshin classes we use the martial arts as a test to see how your energy work is progressing, rather than as a violent sport.

A regular physical fitness regimen will also help your heart, lungs and muscles. As your self-awareness and meditation skills increase you'll begin moving in a constant state of light meditation. A regular fitness plan helps develop your moving meditation skills in addition to making you more fit.

Part of life is dealing with stress, and as we deal with it in one way or another we build up stress knots in our organs and muscles. Many of these knots will connect to a specific energy or memory and when they're released you may find yourself having to deal with that problem or memory again. You can to that gradually, like peeling away the layers of an onion. You can also do it all at once when the Kundalini awakens, like smashing the onion with a big sledgehammer. Fortunately we get to choose how to do it.

Massage, Reiki and Acupuncture

When the stress knots begin to release out of your system you may find it necessary to have some bodywork done. I'm a huge fan of these three as well as chiropractic.

Stress knots are energy. When that energy releases it has to manifest in some way and sometimes it helps to have it massaged out, or to have an acupuncturist go through and balance your energy manually. You'll often experience emotional releases such as crying or laughing during these treatments. It's just the energy releasing and draining out of your system.

Reiki is a form of channeling universal energy through yourself. It can be extremely powerful for healing at all levels and it's an amazing aid to Kundalini awakening as it helps open up and cleanse the chakras. You'll find directions for how to perform a basic Reiki treatment on yourself in later chapter. It's taught as part of the belt requirements in my Hoshin classes. Those interested in learning more about Reiki can download (for FREE!) a complete Reiki Course from my website at www.robertmorgen.com/Reiki1.pdf

The interconnectivity of everything

One of the truly amazing experiences with Kundalini is the feeling of having your *self* disappear and of connecting to everything else. To call it a defining moment in a person's life doesn't do it justice as it literally changes the way you look at and react with everyone and everything around you.

When you can feel *everything* at an energetic level then you realize that thoughts, words and actions have their own energy. Energy follows thought, so when you think about something you do, in fact, create it. It becomes your reality, which is one reason why you'll hear Kundalini and meditation teachers saying over and over again to "be positive".

This is much more than just feeling the universe; it's the literal act of becoming the universe and realizing that the universe *is* you. It's why people who've actually done it have no fear of death. They've experienced the reality of the permanence/impermanence of the universe.

The Law of Reciprocity

When you can feel the complete and total interconnectedness then old sayings like "What goes around, comes around" take on a whole new meaning. We call it The Law of Reciprocity. What you send out *will* be returned to you, so if you send out negative, harmful thoughts or actions then guess what you get back?

It becomes a constant reminder to pay attention to your thoughts and actions. The energy that you put out is the energy that comes back to you, so if you want to be treated with love and compassion then you have to start by treating others with love and compassion.

Using Affirmations

One of the most powerful tools in the universe is one that you can begin using immediately! Affirmations are simple, you can do them anywhere and they don't cost anything.

When you use an affirmation then you are literally making something firm or real for yourself. The subconscious mind (the Id) can't discern between what's real and what isn't, so when you make a positive affirmation like "I deserve LOVE" then the subconscious is there in the background going "Yeah, we do, so where the hell is it. Let's make that happen right now."

The simple way to use these is to identify some part of your life where you feel a lack, and then create the affirmation to convert that lack to abundance.

I'm not going to bother giving you a list of affirmations as you know yourself much better than I do. Instead I'm going to leave a blank place here and as one of your first exercises you can identify 10 areas of your life that you'd like to improve and then create your own affirmation for each. Go ahead and write in the book. It's ok.

I'd like to improve;_____

I deserve/am worthy of_____

I'd like to improve;_____

I deserve/am worthy of_____

I'd like to improve;_____

I deserve/am worthy of_____

I'd like to improve;_____

I deserve/am worthy of_____

I'd like to improve;_____

I deserve/am worthy of_____

I'd like to improve;_____

I deserve/am worthy of_____

I'd like to improve;_____

I deserve/am worthy of_____

I'd like to improve;_____

I deserve/am worthy of_____

I'd like to improve;_____

I deserve/am worthy of_____

I'd like to improve;_____

I deserve/am worthy of_____

Several times a day you should take a few moments and repeat these affirmations to your self until you've created your abundance in these areas. Then come up with some new ones and start all over again.

Avoiding negativity

"Is it possible to have knowledge and yet learn to be free from fear?"
Jiddu Krishnamurti

Just as positive affirmations can bring you abundance, negative affirmations can take it away. Once again the subconscious mind will create whatever you tell it to. When you say things like "I can't do this, it's too hard, I'm not good enough", or some other wussification (see what affirmations do for you? I created a new word just because I could), the subconscious is right there in the background going "Yeah you loser, what were you thinking to even try?" It's just as important to break your old negative habits as it is to replace them with new positive habits.

This is all a part of creating the incremental changes in your life that all add up to BE-ing an enlightened being.

Kundalini and Enlightenment

We always hear about the "Enlightened Master". I find that to be extremely amusing since enlightenment doesn't really exist in and of itself!

Enlightenment only exists as a relative term. There's complete ignorance and lack of awareness on one end of the scale, and Enlightenment on the other. Neither exists independently, but rather as a moment to moment reaction to what's going on around us. Is true enlightenment simply our recognizing the connections that we all have to one another and really treating others as we'd want to be treated, loving others as we should love ourselves?

Awakening the Kundalini or spending a decade in a cave on a mountain doesn't necessarily make one enlightened. Spending every moment actually in the moment and responding to the same divine spark in others that we also have within us possibly does.

Dealing with Attachments

You'll hear a lot about attachments as you begin working with the Kundalini. Part of the process is to divest yourself of your attachments so let's take a look at what that means. Attachments are, in my perception, primarily *ideas* about yourself and others that you hold on to. So don't feel like you have to get rid of the wife or the family pet or sell your favorite putter.

Attachments are part of your ego. Sometimes they may be a part of your learned ego, the super-ego. That's the person you have been taught to be. Other attachments may be a part of your subconscious or Id. You can even have attachments that are holdovers from past lives! (A note about this, the Social Security Administration will NOT accept how screwed up you were in a past life as justification for putting you on a disability pension in this one - just trust me on this.)

As you get deeper into your self-awareness process you'll occasionally find these attachments and have to deal with them. Maybe one of your attachments is to the thought that you should be an Executive in your company by now, so you feel lessened or diminished because you aren't. Maybe you don't fit Hollywood's idea of the ideal weight and you continually feel lessened by your "weight problem". You could become attached to the idea that once you become slim then everything will be ok in your life.

Unfortunately there's not much I can tell you that will help with this. As part of your process you just have to develop the self-awareness to find your attachments and deal with them. This is a different process for everyone.

The Siddhis

"Those who dance are often thought insane by those who can't hear the music"
-George Carlin

Siddhi is an ancient Sanskrit word that means magic. One of the funny (and sometimes annoying) side effects to Kundalini awakening is that you can develop abilities that others don't have and probably don't believe in as the average Westerner doesn't have much first-hand experience with this stuff.

Some of the siddhis will be physical, such as vastly improved health and better balance. In my case I've had huge improvements in my eyesight and my hearing. My balance also improved immensely, partly as a side effect of the release of stress knots and muscle tightness.

Other siddhis may touch on the spiritual or psychic realms. Many Kundalini adepts report an increase in psychic abilities and the tendency to just *know* things (usually seen by non-adepts as the tendency to be a smart-ass). In some cases you may find that you actually channel spirit guides (or ancient wisdom, or whatever you want to call it).

One of the first things that a good Kundalini teacher should tell a student about the siddhis is; "DON'T TALK ABOUT IT!"

(Rule #1 – You don't talk about Kundalini awakening.

Rule #2 – You don't talk about Kundalini awakening.)

The reason is simple. As you get deeper into your self-awareness and then deeper into the awareness of your interconnectivity, you're going to see, feel and experience things that most people never do. If you talk about it then people will think you're seeing and hearing things that they don't. The usual response to that is to give you mind altering drugs and electro-shock therapy to make you 'normal' again.

Having said that, most of us tend to talk about it anyway. Usually, by the time you know enough about it to really talk about it then you have such a strange energy and probably dress weirdly enough that most of the 'normal' people don't really see you.

One of the amazing things about the internet is the ability to form online communities, and this has been a major boon for Kundalini survivors. From 1992 until 2002 I never talked to another human who'd experienced the things I was going through. Now, thanks to the internet, it's possible to go onto a discussion group and ask questions and talk about experiences and just lurk and learn. I've listed several good groups (including mine) in the Resource Section at the end of the book.

Energy attacks and defense

Some recent cartoons have given rise to the 'chi ball' and now I see people talking about this as if it were real, and even worse, spending a lot of effort trying to protect themselves from it.

There *are* some *real* energy attacks and ways to defend against them, however. One of the things that I teach in my Hoshin classes is how to use energy as a tool and send it into various chakras and pressure points. It's not the sort of thing that should be learned from a book or a video. It's also not something that you really need to worry about as the average person can't muster enough concentrated energy to still *their own mind*, so why worry that they might still *your* heart? When I was out at the San Francisco Bujinkan dojo I once saw Dale Seago, a relatively high level Ninjutsu practitioner; knock an attacker's leg out from under him using a secret sword technique. As the attacker ran in, Dale directed a burst of chi into his opponent's leg and the leg just stopped working!

There are also some very simple and safe ways to steal an opponent's energy and strength, but for the most part anyone who can use these techniques will be able to do so against *anyone* who doesn't have a high degree of awareness, so guess what your best defense is. That's right, awareness! The other good thing is that by the time a person develops that much energy they've usually found so many ways to use it more productively that you really don't have to worry about being attacked by them.

The best defense that I can think of, and yes this sounds hokey, is to be completely open and at One. If you have to defend yourself, then let your *self* blend into the rest of the universe. Not only is there nothing to attack, but there's nothing to defend. Think about it til it makes sense. ☺

Sensing Intention

One of the mystical aspects of the martial arts has always been the ability to feel another person's intention. Sensing intention gives a person the ability to be in instant control of a potentially violent encounter, and it's one of the ways we use the martial arts to test our energy work and meditation skills in Hoshin Roshi Ryu.

I'm including this in this book because sensing intention is all about awareness and being in complete control of the moment. It's an ability that's amazingly easy to learn that can also bring new depth to the *non-violence* of your life as it can make you safer and more confident.

A simple explanation of intention

When a person intends to hit you, that intention carries with it a very subtle vibration. Since most people are unaware of this they put off a variety of these subtle vibrations constantly. Have you ever come home to an angry spouse and felt the entire house vibrate with the bad energy? This is exactly the same.

When a person tries to hit you they put off a vibration that you can feel, even with your eyes closed. With training a person can distinguish between the intent to strike and the strike itself as there are subtle differences in the feel of the energy vibrations emanating from the attacker.

In Hoshin class we have a student stand with their eyes closed and then, very slowly, send a punch towards their face with the full intention to make contact. Almost invariably the student will feel the difference in the subtle energies that surround them and their body, seemingly of its own accord, will dodge out of the way. It's fun to see the look of shock on a persons face when they realize what happened and what they felt.

Another exercise is to have a student stand with his back to you, then walk slowly (and silently) forward. The student is to raise a hand when they feel you coming up behind them. You can vary this by thinking angry thoughts and happy thoughts and watch the distance at which you become noticed by the student.

The purpose of teaching a student to feel intention is to empower them in situations that most people find daunting. When you *know* that another person has ill intentions towards you, then you are in control. Depending on the situation you can leave, you can seek a diplomatic solution or you can wait till the future attackers back is turned and hit him with a chair.

While some of these solutions are better than others (Chair Fu should always be the absolute last resort) what's important here is that because of your heightened awareness you weren't taken by surprise when someone attacked you.

For an interesting illustration of using intention and feeling the difference between the intent to strike and the actual strike read Chapter 6 of Dr. Glenn Morris' book *Pathnotes of an American Ninja Master* in which he talks about his experience with the Bujinkan Sword Test.

Spirituality and Religion

"The most damaging phrase in the language is: 'It's always been done that way.'"
- Grace Murray Hopper

It's strange, but some people seem to have conflicts between Spirituality and Religion. I often meet people who say things like "I can't practice Yoga or Zen Meditation because I'm a Christian".

I'm not here to digress into a rant about closed-mindedness or religions which proclaim that you have to "do it our way or roast in hell forever". I just want to take a moment and discuss the differences and why spirituality and religion don't have to be mutually exclusive.

Spirituality is about making a deeper connection to your inner self, getting beyond the politics and dogmas and touching your true inner core. You can do this regardless of which path you follow be it Wicca, Christianity, Judaism, Buddhism or the worship of asbestos ceiling tiles. It's about balancing the Id and the Super Ego and creating the complete sense of harmony with your life and your environment.

Religion on the other hand, has 3 classic purposes (according to my cultural anthropology professor);

1. To answer the otherwise unexplainable questions.

"Where do we come from? Why are we here? What's it all about, etc.?"

2. To provide a sense of continuity between this life and whatever comes after.

"What happens when we die? Where do we go then?"

3. To provide a structure for the laws that we live under.

Every country on the planet has its primary laws based on the rules of their dominant religion.

You can find your spirituality anywhere and there are many people in all of the religions who have done exactly that and have had excellent results and even reached true enlightenment, so I'm not condemning religion. However, there is a tendency in the major religions to try to provide hard, fast *rules* to live under, rather than *principles* to live by and this is where the problems seem to start.

A Rule or Law states that you *must* do it this way, every time. A principle is more variable and depends on the judgment of the person looking at the situation. While rules can be necessary and even good, the reality of our world is that things aren't always so black and white and clearly cut. Living in America today it's easy to see many situations where something is legal under the LAW, but even though it's legal, it's still wrong, according to our accepted mores.

As societies become ever larger it's important to have a clear system of laws to live under, but at the same time it's easy for the charismatic charlatan to sway the masses and then take advantage of them. The ideas of "don't think for yourself, just accept it as it was written and then train your children from birth to believe it also" create an ever growing flock just waiting to be fleeced.

Another way that spirituality conflicts with religion deals with the way that many religions depend on followers who provide a *power base* for the religions (in particular for those in charge of the religions). Free thinkers who are deeply in touch with themselves don't really make the best followers for the theocrats, hence the disdain of some of the spiritual paths by the major religions.

Spirituality tends to be more fluid. It's about knowing yourself and believing in yourself and having the self-awareness to be able to make your own decisions. The interesting aspect of spirituality is that it can greatly enhance whatever religion or philosophy you choose to follow. If there's a religious path that you believe in then your deeper connection to yourself can help you gain insights and wisdom and take you in new directions that can deepen your religious experience.

The religions and spiritual pathways provide different things for different people, and it's important to be as nonjudgmental as possible because we're all in different phases and stages of our development. I try to look at everything as a tool, and different people need different tools. As we progress in learning and living we'll find that our tools change, as well as the way we use them.

The Kundalini Downside

It's not all about cool abilities, increased physical strength and better health, unfortunately. The Kundalini can have a downside for the seeker who doesn't pay attention and follow some simple rules.

Some of the siddhis, especially those in the psychic realms, can cause paranoia, depression and even worse in the unprepared and unknowing. I firmly believe that many of the folks in our asylums who suffer from schizophrenia, epilepsy, depression and paranoia are victims not only of a spontaneous Kundalini awakening, but of a society that doesn't recognize it and has no reality into which the Kundalini fits.

Other side effects that can be annoying (besides insanity) include an increased sexual attraction by the opposite, and even the same, sex. Kundalini is, by definition, sexual energy. It's the primordial energy from which we were all created and once you start boosting it, it can be pretty easy for the opposite sex to feel an unusual attraction to it.

As you balance your chakras (which can be quite a process) you'll possibly go through periods that can only be described as a form of spiritual superiority as you're experiencing things and deities that the average person no longer gets to interact with.

Giving Away Your Stuff

One of the things to remember when the Kundalini awakens is that you'll probably go through some extremely life altering periods. Many teachers advise their students not to make any major changes for at least 6 months after the Kundalini rises. Don't buy, sell or give away anything and don't dump all of your stuff and decide to follow a spiritual path. That's not bad advice, although I go a bit differently with it.

My advice (coming from someone who had a particularly hard time in this period, but who also didn't know anyone else who'd been through it) is to embrace the insanity and roll with it. Give away all your stuff, wear funny clothes and ride the shakti-coaster til the gods all get together and throw you off it. Fortunately today there are relatively easy ways to communicate with others who may be experiencing something similar to you, so you can take time out from lying under a Volkswagen talking to god and go into the library and use the internet. It gives you a bit more freedom to explore.

Chapter 4

Establishing a daily practice

"No man ever became wise by chance".
Seneca

It's important to establish a daily practice and then stick to it, especially in the beginning. This doesn't mean dedicating 12 hours a day to meditation, it just means creating a space in your home where you can take a few minutes and meditate and do the exercises. I advise people to start with some of the basic exercises and devote 10 -20 minutes a day as they develop their physical and mental abilities. Many people quite simply overload themselves and expect too much too soon, then get discouraged when they don't see the results they thought they should see.

In Part 2 of this book you'll find some exercises, ranging from the very basic to the moderately advanced. My advice is to do them in that order, simply because we all have the temptation to jump in over our heads (which can also be a good thing) and overload ourselves.

Getting Started

Set aside a corner in one of your

rooms. You can stock it with whatever accoutrement you wish. Many folks have cushions, candles, incense and a small CD player for music or guided meditation CD's. Use whatever tools and accessories you want to, as there's no right or wrong at this point.

Once you've created your sacred space then all you have to do is use it. Set aside a few minutes each day and begin working through the meditation exercises in Part 2. Don't worry at this point about how long you meditate, just get into the habit of doing it. The effects of meditation are cumulative, so 5 minutes a day everyday is better than 35 minutes once a week.

Eventually you'll get to the point where you don't need any accessories and you can clear your mind and meditate anywhere, at any time, but for now don't worry about that, just create a pleasant, sacred atmosphere and get started.

On Expectation

In the spiritual circles we often hear people talking about doing things "without expectation". It's amazing how often the simple truths are all around us.

When we begin meditation or working towards the Kundalini, we often feel that we should be able to do certain things within a certain time frame. We *expect* to be able to clear our minds and access our deeper abilities. We *expect* to be able to sit for an hour and meditate, or to see auras, or feel other people's chi. Then when it doesn't happen we become disappointed and confused. I can't tell you how important it is to break free of these expectations.

When we let go of expectations and learn to just relax in the moment and just BE, then we are making progress of the most important kind. In the west we tend to be so goal oriented and have a need to see results, but frequently the cumulative effects of meditation aren't noticeable until much later. Meditation is about this moment, about BEing totally in this moment, rather than about who you'll be when you've become a *good* meditator.

The important thing with a regular practice is to just do it. The effects are cumulative and one day you'll look back and see that all those short meditation sessions actually added up.

Part 2

Intro to Meditation

This section is all about actually doing your meditations. The meditations here range from very basic to relatively advanced. Depending on where you are in your studies you may feel that you've progressed beyond some of this, but my advice is to take some time and go back through the basics. One of the benefits of teaching meditation is that I'm constantly running through these basic exercises as I teach them to others, and I can't tell you how helpful that can be. I remember the time before I began teaching when I hardly ever sat through a Brain Scrub session, but then when I began teaching it and sitting through the sessions with my students I found that going back to the basics allowed me to get even deeper into the more advanced exercises.

Chapter 1

Meditation Positions

There are several ways to meditate and depending on your goals you may sit in various positions, stand in various positions or even move and walk around.

Seated Meditation

Sit on a cushion, zafu or a pillow with your spine straight. Don't worry about specific positions such as the full lotus or half lotus, just cross your legs comfortably and let your knees relax.

The purpose of sitting on the cushion is to keep your hips higher than your knees, which helps take the pressure off the muscles that run up through your hips. Keep the spine erect, shoulders back and neck straight and let your hands relax in your lap. Some methods require certain hand positions or mudras, but for now just let your hands relax in a comfortable position in your lap.

In this position your skeletal system should be supporting your body, allowing your muscles to relax completely. Energy doesn't move through tight muscles.

It'll take awhile for you to get used to sitting this way, so just relax and grow into it.

Touch your tongue to the roof of your mouth. Close your eyes and look up towards your third eye (the chakra in your forehead right between your eyes).

Sitting in a chair

Contrary to popular belief, you don't have to be a human pretzel to meditate. Grab a straight-backed chair and sit toward the front of it with your genitals out over the front edge. Keep your feet comfortably flat on the floor, your hips tucked and your spine straight. Let your hands rest in your lap. Touch your tongue to the roof of your mouth. Close your eyes and look up towards your third eye.

Seiza

Seiza is the kneeling position that we see used in many of the Zen temples. You can use this position if you wish, but most people find it extremely uncomfortable for more than a few minutes. In Hoshin Roshi Ryu we use a couple of variations, but they aren't really necessary for Kundalini Awakening.

Standing

When we get into the Chakra exercises we'll be doing some standing meditations using the "Standing Stake" pose from Chi Kung (Qi Qong).

Stand with your feet shoulder width apart, your arms hanging loosely at your sides. Flex your knees slightly. Tuck your hips under slightly and feel your lower spine straighten. Relax your ankles, then your calves, then your thighs, then your buttocks. Let that sense of relaxation flow up your back and across your shoulders and up your neck and on out through the top of your head.

As usual, touch your tongue to the roof of your mouth. Close your eyes and look up towards your third eye.

Moving

As you become more adept at meditation you'll develop the ability to do it while moving. In fact, you'll get to a point where you're in a constant state of light meditation once you learn to access the energy and open up to it. You may already be practicing some of the more formalized forms of moving meditation such as Chi Kung, Tai Chi or yoga.

Anything can be a form of moving meditation, including martial arts, dancing or just playing. What makes it a meditation is your state of mindfulness and your awareness of the moment.

Keeping the tongue up

You'll frequently hear about keeping your tongue on the roof of your mouth. It's extremely important to remember this because when you keep your tongue up you're completing the energy circuit between the Governing and Conception Meridians. Failure to do this can cause energy overloads and actually create some very interesting medical conditions that you'd be better off not experiencing. The doubtful among you can read Dr. Glenn Morris' experiences with this in *Pathnotes of an American Ninja Master.*

The basic position for these exercises is just to touch your tongue to the roof of your mouth just behind your front teeth. Keep your jaw relaxed and your teeth slightly apart.

Your tongue should always be in this position, especially when you begin meditating constantly during your daily life.

As you get deeper into the energy work you can use the other 2 positions, but for now just keep your tongue in the basic position right behind your front teeth.

Color and Sound

Everything is vibration, even color and sound. As you begin these meditation exercises you may find it helpful to choose some light, relaxing music that isn't distracting. Music can have many different effects on us and as you get deeper into the meditations then you'll be able to really enhance your practice with different types of music. There are also a lot of subliminal programs out there that can help reprogram some of your subconscious issues. I've never used any of the subliminal programs and don't know anyone who has, so I truly have no opinion about their effectiveness, but it sounds like a workable idea. It *is* something that I intend to experiment with in the near future though.

Color can also have varying effects. Each chakra has a color associated with it, so you can use color to get in touch with your chakras (more on this in the chakra chapters) or you can just relax and look at the colors that appear in your third eye.

The Healer's Manual by Ted Andrews has some pretty interesting exercises for using colors and sounds. As you build up your sensitivity you'll be able to use and adapt your environment more easily for the energy that you want.

Chapter 2

Breathing

(This exercise is available online as a *FREE Guided Meditation*. Check the website at www.mysticwolfpress.com for download locations)

Breathing is the *most* important part of meditation and Kundalini Awakening. Learning to breathe properly not only helps develop your awareness, it also has numerous health benefits.

From our birth until death we breathe more or less continually, yet for the most part we do it without any awareness of our breath and its effects on us, and believe it or not most people in the western world do it *wrong*!

Breathe in through your nose and draw your breath down into the area just below your navel, allowing your stomach to expand as you breathe (Baby Breath) and filling your lungs entirely with each breath before exhaling through your nose.

Take a moment right now and feel your breath. Pay attention to the air as it flows in through your nostrils and down into your lungs. Don't think about anything or do anything other than just breathe.

1. Are you taking a relatively shallow breath and just filling the upper lobes of your lungs?
2. Does your stomach move out as you breathe?
3. Do you feel the bones of your ribcage expanding and opening with each breath?
For most people the answer to 1 is YES and the answers to 2 and 3 are NO so lets expand this exercise a bit.

Draw your breath down to a point about 2 inches below your navel (the body's center of gravity). When you do this you'll feel your stomach expand and push out in front of you. Most westerners usually keep their stomach pulled in and their chest out, so if you do this you'll have to relax your abdomen. Just take a moment and be aware of your breath as it flows down into your center.

As you inhale and draw your breath down, also let your ribcage expand. You'll feel your floating ribs at the bottom of your ribcage spread and move, and you may get a few pops out of your spine also. Now just take a few moments and breathe this way. Don't think or let your mind wander, just breathe.

If you've never meditated before then congratulations, you just did! It's exactly that simple.

There are many benefits to proper breathing. The extra oxygen in your system means that your heart doesn't have to beat as fast, which lowers your pulse and your blood pressure. Drawing the breath down into your center also helps to massage your internal organs, providing more oxygen to them as well as helping to release the accumulated stresses that build up there. The long term health benefits are immeasurable and have been repeatedly proven for thousands of years.

Breathing is by far the most important part of the Kundalini awakening exercises, although it sounds so simple. Paying attention to the breath is the beginning of opening up your awareness and it's use in meditation is seen in every culture on the planet.

Take some time to practice this, as it's the foundation for everything that comes next. If you have to dedicate your meditation time to breathwork for awhile then that's good, as we all proceed at our own pace.

I recently read a translation of some of Jesus' teachings from the original Aramaic (the language he actually spoke, although he apparently wasn't literate) and it was very interesting to me that in Aramaic they used the same word for *wind, breath* and *spirit*. Those with a Chi Kung background might find it interesting to take another look at the New Testament and insert the word *breath* every time you see the word *spirit*.

Chapter 3

Full Body Awareness

(This exercise is available online as a *FREE Guided Meditation*. Check the website at www.mysticwolfpress.com for download locations)

Once you're comfortable working with your breath it's time to bring the rest of the body in. Continue breathing as I've outlined above. In addition to feeling your breath flow and your stomach and ribs expand, I want you to feel the energy that flows into your body with each breath. For me it feels like a lightness, or a very light feeling. It may feel different for you so take some time here and just open up and feel the energy.

When you draw the energy in can you feel it pooling at your center of gravity just below your belly button? As you breathe just let that pool of energy expand throughout your body. Can you feel it flowing down through your legs and up your back and down your arms? Take some time here and practice this feeling that energy pool expand through your whole body. Later we'll expand it out even further, but for now just let it flow.

This exercise should help you to feel

rejuvenated and refreshed as you're drawing energy from an infinite pool. Do this exercise whenever you're depressed or down, and eventually as you progress you'll learn to do it all the time. It's a habit that you have to grow into.

Awareness and Intention

EVERYTHING is about Awareness and Intention. Now that you've begun to build an awareness of the energy, called Chi, Ki or Prana in some circles, you'll be able to do things with it and move it around in your (and other peoples) body.

We move energy with Intention, and this is a very important fact. EVERYTHING is energy! Our thoughts, our actions, our beliefs, everything around us and everything we see, feel, hear, think and do is energy. *Intention* is what we do with that energy.

We are all connected in a vast energy pool that encompasses everything that is, was and will be. It doesn't matter whether a person believes in it or can feel it; they still have the ability to affect it. How many times have you seen a person with a negative attitude who continually draws more negative reactions to himself? He's broadcasting his intentions through his attitudes with the result that he becomes a human crap magnet, drawing in all the negative feelings and emotions and experiences.

The other side of this is the continually

positive person who always approaches everything from a positive attitude. This doesn't mean that everything always goes the way he wants it, but if you'll watch you'll see that even the bad times provide fuel for his growth and he tries to take every bad experience as a lesson to help improve himself.

Just as our thoughts can influence Chi subconsciously, so can they move it around in our body. *Energy follows thought,* so when you think about moving energy then it will actually go where you send it. The important thing here is to stay out of its way. Energy moves in a spiral and at its own speed, so don't try to micro-manage it, just let it flow.

Take some time and do the Full Body Awareness exercise again, and this time feel the energy go where you send it. You can also play with this a bit. Send it down to your feet, now bring it back to your center and this time just send it down to your left foot, now your right. Now send it up to your head, and down to your left elbow.

The next time you're stuck in traffic, or impatiently waiting in line at the Motor Vehicles Office, just relax and start to play with this. Isn't this a neat toy?

Chapter 4

Basic Exercises

Now that you've begun to develop the ability to move energy around in your body there are some things that you can do with it. The following exercises range from pretty simple to pretty complicated, but as you develop your abilities you'll eventually find that you can do them all at once and effortlessly. It can take anywhere from a few weeks to a few years to develop this ability, so remember what I said about expectations.

You'll eventually be able to remember how to do these exercises by memory, and then after that you'll get to the point where you just do them without having to think about them. In the beginning it may be helpful to have a partner read the exercises to you or you can order the CD Set that goes with this book at www.robertmorgen.com.

Grounding

Grounding will always be an important skill, no matter how advanced you become, so take the time to learn this now and to be able to do it effortlessly.

Stand in the "Standing Stake" pose described above. Go through the breathing and Full Body Awareness exercises. Visualize roots growing from your feet down through the core of the earth, just like a tree. In later meditations you can add some variety by seeing the roots flow down to a large crystal at the earth's core. Depending on the effect you want you can vary the crystals and access different energies, but that obviously beyond the scope of the exercise at this point.

As you inhale feel the energy of the earth being drawn up through your roots and up through your body and out through the top of your head.

On your exhale, let that energy drop back down through your body and feel all the accumulated stress of your life flow out with it and back down through your roots and into the earth. Feel your muscles relax as the stress flows out. This is a good way to release all your stresses, fears, angers and feelings of inadequacy. Repeat this exercise for awhile, as many times as necessary to clean yourself out.

There's nothing wrong (and a lot of benefit) to stopping at this point and just doing these exercises that I've gone over up to this point, until they become completely effortless. Whenever you feel yourself becoming stressed or angry learn to take a moment and ground yourself and let those feelings just flow out.

Progressive Relaxation

Progressive Relaxation is easy to do

and you can do it anywhere and anytime.

Assume your meditation position of choice (I like the half-lotus on a zafu) and go through all the exercises I've covered up to this point. Just take a moment and feel the relaxed energy that you should have after grounding and releasing all your stress. Are you ready to get deeper into this feeling?

Feel the energy that flows up through your roots and into your feet. Make fists with your feet by curling your toes in as far as you can until it hurts, then relax. Let that relaxed feeling flow from your toes back over your feet and feel them relax.

As you inhale draw that relaxed feeling up over your ankles and feel them relax completely. On the exhale let any residual stress flow back out and down through the earth.

On your next inhale draw that relaxed feeling back up over your calves, letting them relax after walking all day.

Draw that relaxed energy up over your thighs with the next inhale. They're the biggest muscles in the body, so let them relax and rest now.

As you inhale feel that relaxed feeling flow up over your hips and buttocks. Feel the stress bleed away. We store a lost of stress here, so take a moment and let this area relax.

Draw that relaxed feeling up over your stomach and lower back. Feel the muscles in your back relax and feel your stomach move with your inhale.

Bring the energy up over your chest and the middle of your back. Feel your heart area expand with the relaxed energy and feel all the accumulated stress in between your shoulder blades release and flow out and back down with your exhale.

Draw the feeling of relaxation up over your shoulders and neck. Feel any residual tension flow out with your exhale.
Let that relaxed energy flow up and over your head. Let the muscles of your face and those at the base of your skull relax.

Just sit here and feel this relaxed body that you have. Remember this feeling as its how you should feel all the time. Tense muscles store energy, which means that your energy isn't flowing through you, but rather sticking in certain places in your body.
When your muscles are relaxed then your energy flows unimpeded and is continually renewed, leaving you feeling much lighter and more refreshed.

The Brain Scrub

The Brain Scrub is designed to help you overcome the "monkey mind" which leaps and bounces around from subject to subject in an uncontrolled manner. After mastering this exercise you'll be able to instantly clear and calm your mind in any situation, allowing you to focus completely on any subject.
First hit the position, as described

above. Take a moment to relax and let your breathing soften.

As you inhale focus on the number 1. Hold your focus and exhale.

On the next inhale focus on the number 2 and so on until you get to 10.

The purpose here is to focus entirely on the numbers and not allow any other thoughts to intrude.

DO NOT beat yourself up with this exercise! Our minds are constantly at work and the untrained mind will bounce from thought to thought continually (monkey mind) and even during this exercise you'll have other thoughts arise.
The key is not to *attach* to any of those thoughts. When other thoughts arise just let them evaporate like a wisp of smoke, passing unheeded through your consciousness and on out of your head.

Your goal is to count from 1 to 10 without attaching to any intruding thoughts, and if you do find yourself thinking of anything other than your target number then go back to one and start over.

This exercise is invaluable for learning to control your mind, and even seasoned meditators will find it useful to go back and practice occasionally.

Drawing Energy

During various exercises we'll be drawing energy in through our chakras, into our organs and even through the entire area of our skin. Drawing energy into yourself is fairly easy to do and simply requires a heightened sense of self-awareness to feel.

To begin drawing energy just take a moment and focus on your breathing. Feel your breath as it flows in through your nostrils and down to your Dan Tien, the area two finger-widths below your belly button. Feel the chi as it flows in with your breath down to your Dan Tien. Take a few breaths and let the energy build up and spread through your body.

Now, as silly as it sounds, imagine a nose or an opening that covers your heart chakra, just over your sternum. Remember what it feels like when you draw the chi in through your nostrils? As you inhale let the 'nose' over your heart chakra 'inhale' chi directly into your heart. It may take awhile to really feel this, so don't be worried if it doesn't seem to come easily. As you exhale let any stress or unhappiness in your heart chakra flow down through your legs and deep into the earth.

Take some time and practice 'inhaling' energy this way. As you get comfortable with it you'll be able to draw chi into yourself in many different ways. Below are some sample exercises that you can experiment with. You'll probably come up with some others on your own as the possibilities here are literally endless.

Chakra Breathing– We'll get deeper into this in the Chakra Chapters, but you can draw energy into any of your chakras at any time just like we did for the heart chakra.

Energizing your organs– This can be a lot of fun and really help strengthen your immune system and improve your overall health. It's also an exercise in using intention to send energy where you want it to go.

Take a moment and relax as we did above. On your inhale draw chi into your Liver. Don't worry if you don't know exactly where your liver is, you don't have to. Just intend for relaxing, healing energy to flow into your liver as you inhale, and then draw it in. On your exhale let the stresses and built up energies flow out of your liver and down into the earth. Can you feel the lightness and relaxation? The next time you find yourself becoming angry do this exercise.

You can run chi into any of your organs exactly the same way. The infusion of energy will help cleanse your organs and release bound stresses and memories, so you may find yourself having some unexpected emotional releases also as that energy has to go somewhere once it's released.

Relaxing Stress Knots out of your muscles– Whenever you feel a stress knot building up in your muscles just draw energy directly into the knot on the inhale and let the stress flow down into the earth on your exhale. As an exercise in awareness you can take some time and just choose a body part at random and draw energy into it.

Improve your eyesight and hearing– I've personally experienced some radical healing in both my eyesight and hearing just by drawing more chi into my eyes and ears. At an age when my eyes should be getting worse I actually have gotten to the point where I only wear my glasses when I'm working on the computer or watching a movie.

Drawing energy from trees, rocks and plants– Sit with your back to a tree or better yet face it and wrap your arms around it. Relax and spend a few moments practicing feeling your own energy. Expand your awareness to the tree. Can you feel the rough bark against your skin and hear the rustle of wind in the leaves and branches. Can you smell it? Can you feel the energy from it? Create a circuit with the tree. As you inhale feel the energy from the tree flow into you. As you exhale let your energy flow into the tree. Let your friends who haven't experienced this laugh at you for being a 'tree hugger'. Experiment with this with other plants as well as rocks and crystals. Do they all feel the same? Can you tell the difference between tree species based on the feel of their energy? Can you differentiate between different crystals based on their energy? You could keep yourself occupied indefinitely in the backyard with this exercise.

Drawing energy is something that you can do at any time, any place. As you get better at it and more comfortable with it you'll also be able to develop more control over your emotions and your physical responses by using variations on the exercises above. Don't be afraid to play with this and experiment with the healing energies as this is all about building up your personal catalog of feelings and experiences.

The Secret Smile

The Secret Smile is one of Dr. Glenn Morris' exercises and he wrote about it in his book *Pathnotes of an American Ninja Master*. Those of us who teach his martial art form, Hoshin Roshi Ryu, also teach this regularly in our classes. This is really a fairly easy exercise and I can't recommend it strongly enough. Energy flows better through a relaxed and happy body and you should get in the habit of making this a regular part of your practice.

Hit the meditation position of choice. Take some time to do the grounding exercise and relax your breathing. Put a smile on your face and keep it there.

To start the Secret Smile first clench your toes as tightly as possible, until it begins to hurt. Relax them and feel the feeling that follows a kind of relaxed, happy, glad not to be tightly clenched feeling. Pull that feeling up across your feet, then up your ankles and up along your calves. Feel it rise up across your knees, then over your thighs and across your hips. Feel the muscles relax as you do this. Draw the feeling up your spine and up over your head and down to the point where your tongue touches the roof of your mouth just behind your front teeth. Mix the relaxed feeling with the saliva in your mouth and then swallow it down and feel it drop down through your body relaxing it as it goes.

Think about a time when you did something well. It can be any event you wish, but think of a time when you did something really right and everyone knew it. Take out the event and just keep the feeling of it. Take that feeling down to your toes and then pull that feeling up across your feet, then up your ankles and up along your calves. Feel it rise up across your knees, then over your thighs and across your hips. Draw the feeling up your spine and up over your head and down to the point where your tongue touches the roof of your mouth just behind your front teeth. Mix the good, competent feeling with the saliva in your mouth and then swallow it down and feel it drop down through your body charging it with the good feeling it as it goes. Let it mix with the first one.

Think about a time when you laughed, a good deep belly laugh that you couldn't control or stop. Now take out the reason for the laughter, but keep the feeling of it. Take that laughing feeling down to your toes and then pull that laughter up across your feet, then up your ankles and up along your calves. Feel it rise up across your knees, then over your thighs and across your hips. Draw the feeling up your spine and up over your head and down to the point where your tongue touches the roof of your mouth just behind your front teeth. Mix the happy, laughing feeling with the saliva in your mouth and then swallow it down and feel it drop down through your body feeling your body laughing it as it goes. Let it mix with the others.

Think about a time when you were in love, truly, completely, 100%, head over heels, swept off your feet in love. Take out the person or people. Take that feeling down to your toes and then pull it up across your feet, then up your ankles and up along your calves. Feel it rise up across your knees, then over your thighs and across your hips. Draw the feeling up your spine and up over your head and down to the point where your tongue touches the roof of your mouth just behind your front teeth. Mix the loving feeling with the saliva in your mouth and then swallow it down and feel it drop down through your body charging it with complete, unconditional love. Let it mix with the others.

Think about the best orgasm you ever had. Take out the person or people and just keep the feeling of the orgasm. Take that feeling down to your toes and then pull that feeling up across your feet, then up your ankles and up along your calves. Feel it rise up across your knees, then over your thighs and across your hips. Draw the feeling up your spine and up over your head and down to the point where your tongue touches the roof of your mouth just behind your front teeth. Mix the feeling with the saliva in your mouth and then swallow it down and feel it drop down through your body charging it with the good feeling it as it goes. Let it mix with the others.

Feel the combination of the energies now and feel the combined energies swirling around down at your feet. Take the feelings down to your toes and then pull that feeling up across your feet, then up your ankles and up along your calves. Feel it rise up across your knees, then over your thighs and across your hips. Feel the happy, relaxed, loving, competent, sexual energy as it flows up your spine and up over your head and down to the point where your tongue touches the roof of your mouth just behind your front teeth. Mix the combined feelings with the saliva in your mouth and then swallow it down and feel it drop down through your body and then let it flow up again to the top of your head, and then drop down to your feet. Play with this awhile, run it as often as you can. This is how you should feel all the time, relaxed, happy, loved and sexy. As you get better at this you'll be able to run it continuously.

The Microcosmic Orbit

In his excellent book *Awaken Healing Energy through the Tao;* Mantak Chia goes into great detail on the Microcosmic Orbit. We teach it in Hoshin Roshi Ryu also. Use this exercise to get started, but *get his book* and get deeper into it.

The purpose with this deceptively simple exercise is to begin drawing your chi up your spine and then back down the front of your body. When you do this you energize your entire body and your internal organs, increasing your health and building up your ability to move more and more energy. All we're doing here at the basic level is drawing the energy up from the perineum the spine to the top of the head and then letting it fall back down the front of our body to the perineum again. Be sure to keep your tongue up to connect the meridians.

Basic Practice

Sitting in a chair or on a cushion, go through the grounding and the Secret Smile. As you inhale clench the PC muscle in your perineum (kegels) and let the energy flow up your spine to the top of your head. Let it flow over the top of your head and then drop down the front of your body to your perineum on the exhale.

As you inhale contract your PC muscles and your sphincter and feel the rush of energy up your spine. This part can take a bit of practice and my advice is begin by only doing a few contractions at a time and then building up the number of contractions as you practice.

At the most basic level that's all there is to it. As you begin to play with this and experiment then you can try running the orbit between various chakras also.

If you feel like you're building up too much heat in your head (headaches, hot forehead) then you can reverse the flow and just run the orbit backwards.

Begin to get into the habit of running the orbit all the time. This gets easier as you become more comfortable with it and learn to stay out of the way of the energy and just let it flow.

Intermediate Practice

The next stage is called the Macrocosmic Orbit and it includes your arms and legs. You should be to the point where you can run the basic orbit at any time, even while at work and during the day as you go about your life. Going from the Microcosmic Orbit to the Macrocosmic Orbit is simple because by now you've figured out the hard parts and just need to expand your orbit.

Draw earth energy up the *front* of your legs as far as the first chakra, then up your spine on the inhale while doing your sphincter contractions. After you pull the energy over the top of your head let it drop back down the front of your body to the perineum and then down the *back* of your legs into the earth. Seen from the side this looks like a figure 8 with an open bottom.

As you draw up the front of your legs also pull energy up the *back* of your arms to the midpoint of your back between your shoulder blades. At this point it combines with the energy coming up your spine and then rises up over your head. It can take some practice to coordinate your breathing with drawing the energy up your arms and legs. It's perfectly fine if you practice these separately and just draw up your legs for awhile before adding in your arms.

On the exhale let your energy drop down the front of your body. When it reaches your heart chakra let it split and let the energy run down the front of your arms as well as the front of your body. Let it flow out your fingers and down to the earth and let the energy flowing down the front of your body go through the perineum and then down the back of your legs, into the earth.

It may take awhile to build your coordination with this so don't get discouraged. This is a good exercise for clearing stagnant energy out of your arms and legs and energizing your entire body. Keep at it til you can get out of the way of the process and just let it flow all the time. You'll reach a point where you can stop *trying* to do it and just let it happen.

Skin Breathing

Skin Breathing is an excellent full body awareness exercise that also helps strengthen your bones, among other things. It's out of the "Marrow Washing and Tendon Changing" school of Chi Kung.

To begin, first take a moment to do the grounding exercise and progressive relaxation exercises. Pay attention to your breathing. On the inhale draw energy into your body as described in the 'Drawing Energy' section, except that instead of drawing chi into a specific organ or muscle we're going to draw it in through the entire surface area of our skin.

This is a relatively advanced exercise. If you have trouble feeling the surface of your skin over your entire body all at once then just take a more manageable chunk such as your head or hands to start with.

As you inhale feel the chi flow in through your skin and deep into your bones. On your exhale feel any stresses or problems flow down through your arms and legs and deep into the earth. Practice this until you can feel the energy flowing into every square inch of skin over your entire body.

Exercises to Open the Meridians

My buddy Brian Earnest sent me these exercises to use in my Hoshin class, and then we videotaped him leading the class through them and turned that into the first episode of the Sustainable Living TV Series. I'm not going into a huge amount of detail with this one since the video is available as a *free download* off the internet. You can get it at

www.mysticwolfpress.com/HarmonyTV

Tao Yin (Taoist Yoga)
By Brian Earnest

Tao-Yin exercises help your internal life force, or Chi, to circulate more freely, for the purpose of refreshing, attuning, adjusting and regenerating your personal energy. All the Tao-Yin movements are based on ancient spiritual development. Taoist Yoga floor postures stretch the difficult-to-reach psoas muscle, calm the mind, open energy channels, and relieve stress.

An important aspect of Tao-Yin is that it has alternating phases of activity and relaxation. During the relaxation phase you will learn to feel and gently guide the Chi flow to specific areas of your body. You will learn to absorb the nutrition from the air and the surrounding energy so you can open each cell to the fresh vitality of the universal force. This practice will help you relieve any energy stagnancy.

Most Tao Yin (or Do-In in Japanese) or Meridian exercises are directly or indirectly related to energizing the flow of electromagnetic currents through the meridians, and in that sense it is not necessary to put special emphasis on exercises for the meridians alone. However, we can use certain exercises especially for the purposes of extending the meridians to activate and release energy flow from any stagnation which may be caused by improper diet, improper posture, or various unnatural daily activities.

MERIDIAN EXERCISES:

There are 12 major meridians for the circulation of Qi on each side of the body in the "traditional meridian system." These 12 meridians are grouped into 6 Yin/Yang pairs in relation to basic life functions.

In addition to the 12 major meridians, in traditional Chinese Medicine, there are 8 extra meridians which are special pathways for the Qi travel. The Conception Vessel and the Governor Vessel are exceptional among the extra meridians in that they also have independent functions and points which are located on the center line in the front and along the back of the body's centerline (independent points are acupuncture points which belong to one meridian. All the regular meridians have independent points, but most of the extra meridians do not. Meridians without independent points share points which belong to other meridians). The most exceptional feature of these 2 meridians is that they regulate the flow of energy in all of the regular meridians. The Conception and Governor Vessels are said to respectively serve as reservoirs of Qi for the Yin/Yang meridians.

Open CV (Conception Vessel)

While bending back holding behind bottom.

The lines of tension produced along the center line of the abdomen are the Conception Vessel. This is the flow of Qi which regulates all the Yin meridians. The conception vessel is a meridian running along the center line on the front of the body which has at least 24 main independent points beginning at the perineum and ending right in the middle of the lower jaw.

Open GV (Governing Vessel)

Bend forward holding behind bottom at top of thighs.

The line of tension which forms down the center of your back is the Governor vessel. The Governor vessel has at least 28 main independent points and begins at the tip of the tailbone and goes up and around the crown of the head to the end up at the midpoint of the upper jaw. The tension along the Governor vessel is felt most strongly when you inhale.

There are 12 major meridians which can be divided into 6 pairs according to Yin (quiet energies) and Yang (active energies).

For best results; during these 6 Meridian exercises we should hold the postures at their extreme extended point for the duration of at least two breath cycles.

This serves for the extension of the meridians as well as the acceleration of energy flow, resulting in the release of stagnation and disorders along the meridians and muscles.

1. Lung/Large Intestine "A" (bend over, look to the heels, push hands over head and up)

2. Stomach / Spleen "B" (Lean back from Seiza)

3. Heart / Small Intestine "C" (Pull forehead towards the floor and try to touch Toes while holding them with the hands and opening the "Gau" groin, feet and heels pressing together)

4. Bladder / Kidney "D" (Legs stretched out heels touching, bend forward and reach)

5. Heart Constrictor (Governor) / Triple Heater Meridians "E" (Sit in ¼ or ½ Lotus position and cross arms one over the other so hands are cupping over opposite knees, bend over and touch forehead to center at crease of arm)

6. Gallbladder / Liver "F" (Both Legs are stretched/extended out to either side. Spread out as far as comfortable. Keep knees straight so that backs of legs touch the floor. Reach up and then out to either side and lean to one side and then the other).

Important Points:

The real purpose of these Six Basic Meridian Exercises is not to attain the flexibility of a gymnast or ballerina. The most important goal is to find the best position in which you can feel the resistance or a tingling sensation coming from the line of tension forming along the meridians.

The main objective here is to get a feeling for what it really is like to relax by releasing Qi and allowing tension to dissipate. Start out doing only two reps for each exercise and one or two complete breath cycles while in each posture. Increase the reps and breath cycles over time. Use slow and deliberate breath patterns. Always keep your attention on your breathing and be sensitive to how your body is responding to each exercise.

Just relax after completion. Relax for a while on your back with your eyes closed in an "X" position (the kind of position we got into when lying in the snow to make snow angels, also called the "Corpse" position in Yoga. Keep the eyes closed and feel for any bodily sensations. Become entirely detached from the external world. When you do this, your mind will begin to tune in to any internal events of your body. You may begin feeling various sensations like tingling or buzzing in the ears, eyes or along the course of the meridians which can be regarded as "Energy Flow." These sensations, instead of issuing from conscious awareness, have their origins in the inner workings of your body.

These meridian exercises should not be viewed merely as a way of stretching and limbering muscles and joints. Stretching in this context does not refer just o lengthening or pulling something apart, but is rather an act of extending or expanding which liberates the energy lying latent within you. These exercises would serve as a form of physical expression to release, through the act of stretching, those things which you have been holding inside. These exercises are an opportunity to get in touch with your body and give expression to your inner being through movement.

Bibliography:
Zen Imagery Exercises, Meridian exercises for wholesome living
By *Shizuto Masunaga*

The Book of Do In
By *Michio Kushi*

The Book of Shiatsu
By *Paul Lundbreg*

Attune your Body with Dao-In
By Master Hua-Ching Ni

Part 3

Connecting to your Inner Self

Chapter 1

Feeling Energy

If you've been doing the exercises that I've described then by this point you've probably had some interesting experiences with feeling your own internal energy and drawing energy into your body. Now we're going to work with feeling external energy. As you progress with this you'll not only be able to feel your own energy, but the energy of the people and things around you.

The following exercises will help you feel your aura, the external energy field that surrounds everything. Everything on the planet is made up of various particles held together by energy, and you can feel and even manipulate that energy with practice.

Exercise 1 – Building an energy ball
Rub your hands together briskly as if trying to warm them on a cold day. Doing this increases the sensitivity.

Hold your hands in front of you about 6 inches apart. Now move them away from each other until they are about 8-12 inches apart, and then move them back to 2-3 inches apart, just like a fisherman describing the sizes of the fish he caught. As you continue doing this can you feel a ball or energy building up between your hands? It feels like a thickness in the air between your hands, or a pressure between them.

Play with this exercise a bit. See how big you can make the energy ball. Is one hand more sensitive than the other? Can you turn your hands over and do it with the backs of your hands?

Exercise 2 – Waving the energy

Hold your left hand upright in front of you with your palm facing to the right. Wave your right fingertips slowly up and down in front of your left hand, but without touching it. Can you feel the motion of your right hand across the surface of your left palm? Switch hands and do it again. Does it feel different with the other hand? Is one hand more sensitive?

Exercise 3 – Feeling the aura

Hold your hands out in front of you at arms length, palms in. Now move your awareness down to your palms and slowly move your palms in towards your body. Remember the way it felt when you made the energy ball between your palms? Can you feel the same sort of thickness or pressure as your palms move in towards your body?

With a partner practice moving your hands slowly towards them. Can you feel their aura? Can your partner feel your hands as you move towards them?

Have your partner stand about 12-15 feet away. Now walk slowly towards them. Can you sense their aura as you walk up to them? Can they feel you? As you get deeper into this you'll be able to play with intention and emotions also, but for now just concentrate on feeling the aura.

Some games that you can play with this;

Have your partner stand a few feet away and think angry thoughts. Can you feel a difference in their energy? How about when they think happy thoughts?

Some people have no trouble at all with this while others aren't as empathic and take awhile to learn to feel it. As usual this is all about building up your own personal catalog and learning how things feel.

Chapter 2

Chakra Diagnosis

Have your partner stand upright but relaxed. Stand with both your hands held above their head. Slowly bring your hands down until you can feel the thickness or pressure of their crown chakra. This can vary on everyone. How far above their head did you feel it?

Move your hands down to their 3rd eye with one hand in front of their forehead and one hand behind their head. Move your hands out and then slowly back towards them until you can sense the energy of their chakra. Did you feel a difference between the front and back? Did you sense the front and back at different distances, was one of them noticeably further out than the other? Did it feel like your hands were pushed out away from the chakra?

Do this again at the Throat Chakra, then at the Heart Chakra, Solar Plexus, and Dan Tien. Don't actually touch them physically; just feel the energy of their chakras.

For the Root Chakra let your hands go down to just above your partners knees and feel the energy over that entire area.

This exercise can be a lot of fun, especially as you learn more about the Chakra system and what it means when you can feel the energy. It's extremely easy to do and anyone with a basic level of awareness can do it fairly quickly as it's just feeling energy.

With practice you can build up the sensitivity to be able to sense another persons chakras without going through the whole diagnosis. When you build up the sensitivity you may even be able to use your own chakras as antennae to *feel* other people's chakras. It sounds weird, but it can be extremely amusing to sit in public (bookstores are good for this) and feel the people that walk by.

When you learn about the chakras then what you sense can be extremely useful for learning about the folks you're dealing with and give you insights into their personalities and their possible actions/reactions. This can be somewhat akin to magic as these abilities are not only misunderstood, but scoffed at and disbelieved by most of western society.

Chapter 3

Seeing the Aura

Just as you can feel energy, a lot of people can also see it. Seeing the aura doesn't seem to be something that everyone can do and those who do seem to have wildly varying abilities. I've known healers who could look at you and say things like "Oh you're blocking some energy here" just because of what they see in your aura while others can just barely see it.

Personally I'm more of an empath and while I can feel energy from across the room I don't see it that well. This is something that you can play with and if you can do it then it's just another cool tool in the toolbox.

Seeing the aura is a matter of taking your eyes slightly out of focus. If you've ever been able to see those holographic picture-in-a-picture things then you shouldn't have any trouble seeing auras as you do exactly the same thing with your eyes. The first time I was at a seminar and this topic came up I had no luck whatsoever with seeing the auras of the other folks in the seminar. That night I went over to the bookstore and grabbed a bunch of the holograph picture books and sat there til I could relax my eyes and see them. The next day when I went back for the rest of the seminar I didn't have any trouble at all seeing the auras of the other attendees.

Have your training partner stand in front of a light-colored wall in a dimly lit room. Have your partner hold one finger in front of their face about 6 inches out from their chin. Now focus your eyes on their finger, not their face. Have them remove their finger but keep looking at the same spot, you'll have to relax your eyes a bit to do this. Now using that same relaxed vision, if you look at them you should be able to see what looks like a little line that runs all around them a couple of inches out from their body. The next layer out is even more faint and may have colors associated with it. The different meanings of the colors vary widely depending on who you're talking to. My advice in this area is to open up your awareness and see for yourself which colors seem to be associated most often with which types of people and their behaviors.

Play with this a bit. Does their aura change when they think happy thoughts? Sad thoughts? Angry thoughts?

Some people can see auras instantly and others have to work at it. Don't be too put out if it takes awhile.

Chapter 4

Finding your 'Inner Gods'

I like the idea of *Gods* but personally don't put much effort or work into worshiping any that I've heard of so far. I frequently see the word Namaste tossed around ("the Divine in me recognizes and honors the Divine in you") and I really like that even though I don't use it much.

Most of the Great Teachers (Christ, Buddha, Mohamed, Krishna, etc.) have been adamant that the Divine or Holy Spirit lives within each of us and that we can all access it without the need for priests, popes, clerics, pastors, televangelists or other middle men. This goes along with the commonly heard "Everything you need is already inside you" attitude that I've learned to believe in.

Some people feel the need to personify their deities and even have different deities for different actions, causes, days of the week, etc. Hence the vast pantheons in some of the religions. I think that's great also. Your mind can bring reality to any thought or concept, so if you want to worship Our Lady Of The Dirty Laundry then by all means feel free and don't ever let anyone tell you she isn't real. I personally really enjoy some of the 'honoring the sacred feminine' rituals. I tend to argue that some of the strictures placed on women in the larger religions go back to men who are afraid of their feminine energies and represents an imbalance in their basic dualities.

You should see your inner deities from any viewpoint that you wish, in other words. Feel free to ritualize, sanctify, idolize and worship them in any way you see fit as it's extremely important to have FAITH when you're on the Kundalini road. It doesn't matter what you choose to have faith in, just as long as you're able to relax and listen to the inner voices and trust that they are taking you in the directions in which you're supposed to go.

My personal feeling here is that you should identify with the happy, positive and beautiful aspects of your inner deities and always strive to remember and honor them in every moment of your life. Your inner deities are part of the same energy that everyone else's inner deities are made of, so by honoring yourself you should also be honoring them and vice versa.

Chapter 5

Complete Self Acceptance

One of the most important parts of Personal Mastery is Self Acceptance. This is much more than the usual self esteem issues that we hear about, although that's a part of it.

Self Acceptance is about accepting yourself completely, exactly as you are RIGHT NOW. For most of us this isn't as easy as it should be. We've been taught that we have to achieve certain things or be certain things, and that we shouldn't feel satisfied with who we are until we've done so.

In reality we're NEVER finished as there will hopefully always be more to learn and new ways to grow. So when, exactly, are we supposed to feel good about ourselves?

Popular culture would have you believe that all you need to feel good about yourself is the right car, or the right clothes, or the right beer. In fact many of our culture's self-esteem problems are *intentionally created* by the media and the businesses that advertise there. How often have you seen an ad and thought "I really *need* to update my style", or "I really *need* a new car"? Do you really? Hey, maybe sometimes we do. I have to admit that my habit of wearing sweatpants, t-shirts and sandals wouldn't go over well when making advertising sales calls for the videos or magazine, and I do in fact, really *need* a good car.

As usual the question in our society is 'how much do we really *need*'? For instance, I don't need Armani suits to sell advertising for a holistic magazine, and I can get by very well with a reliable older car.

The difference here is the word *need* versus the word *want*. We're taught that we *need* certain things to feel good about ourselves, and that's the key issue. I don't care if you buy a new Mercedes 3 times a week if that's what you want to do and you can afford it.

However, if you feel like you need to buy or do *anything* in order to feel good about yourself then that's an issue that needs to be addressed.

Self Acceptance is about FREEDOM. It's the freedom to be happy with who you are and not be a slave to the needs that we're taught to believe in. It's the freedom to look at yourself in the mirror and love and accept the person you see looking back and the freedom to be happy to be in your own skin.

True self acceptance is one of the transformational moments in our lives. It doesn't mean that there aren't things you'd like to change, or have new directions you'd like to grow. It simply means that you've accepted yourself, with all your warts and ugly spots, and now you can start moving in the positive directions needed for your life.

It's also the key to having the freedom to accept others exactly as they are. The most important person that you can love is yourself. Have you ever seen someone who gives up their entire lives to help others, yet destroy their own health and welfare in the process? Everything is connected and One, which means that anything that you can see, feel or imagine is a part of you also, with all the balances that apply.

For instance, a person who only takes care of himself, with no regard for others, is no less imbalanced than someone who devotes his entire life to care for others at the expense of himself.   The key here, once again, is the word NEED. It's all about the motivation that drives them.

Some of those so intent on self-sacrifice are driven by need. They *need* to help others to make up for their own inadequacies, or to make up for the bad things they feel that they've done, or whatever other reasons drive them. Yet if they truly accepted themselves then would they feel the need to sacrifice themselves in order to help others? Wouldn't they see helping others as an extension of helping themselves, rather than as a way to make themselves feel better about who they are?

A balanced person sees helping others as a normal, compassionate thing to do, rather than as something to do to make up for their own lack in some area. It's the Law of

Reciprocity again, by helping others we help ourselves, by encouraging others to grow we also grow in the process. By accepting ourselves exactly as we are, we can also accept others exactly as *they* are, and that's the beginning of unity.

Part 4

The Chakras

Chapter 1

The 7 Primary Chakras

Chakra is a Sanskrit word that means 'wheel' and it refers to the spinning energy centers on our body. A chakra isn't really a physical part of our body although with practice you can feel them pretty easily.

These energy centers affect the way our body functions on all planes as well as store memories and feelings. There is some pretty persuasive evidence that we can even store 'left-over' feelings and memories from former lives. Occasionally these hold-overs can have adverse effects on our current lives.

During a Kundalini awakening you'll go through a period of chakra cleansing and balancing. This period can (as in my case) last for years, although that obviously varies from person to person. This cleansing is part of what many Kundalini teachers refer to when they say that the Kundalini "breaks the wheel of Karma".

Many volumes have been written on the study of chakras and I'm not going to try to recreate that here. Rather than an exhaustive study I'm going to give you enough to get you started and to begin exploring your chakra system.

Those of you who wish to get deeper into the study of chakras (and it's pretty fundamental) are advised to find a copy of

Cyndi Dale's excellent book *New Chakra Healing* as well as my upcoming *Inner Space* series on the Chakras.

When most people mention chakras they are actually talking about the seven primary chakras that run up a person's center line. These seven primary chakras affect our lives on many different levels and a clear understanding of them and what they do is extremely helpful on your quest for self-awareness.

The Japanese based martial arts usually have only 5 chakras; Earth, Water, Fire, Wind and the Void. The Void actually encompasses the top three chakras seen in other systems. In order to avoid too much confusion I've avoided giving all the names from all the various languages that usually associate with chakras.

The chakras have both a front side and a back side. Each side deals with different aspects of your life. The Simple charts below will give you some specifics about it. Most of the information in the charts came from *New Chakra Healing* and deal with the front side of the chakra. My upcoming *Inner Space* series goes into much more detail.

1st Chakra

The First Chakra is also known as the Root or Earth Chakra.

Location	Perineum, groin
Color	Red
Key Word	Awareness
Descriptors	Images of a snake, dragon or "holy fire".
Source Of	Passion; raw, primal feelings, rage, terror, joy, survival energy
Seat of	The will to live
Problems	Root of addictions, compulsions, sexual dysfunction, nervous disorders, money, career and finance issues
Contains	Roots, family values, heritage. Programming affecting basic needs such as sex, money, love, food, air, housing, etc.
Physical Communication Style	Communicates physical/emotional needs through aches and pains, physical awareness, touch, smell, vibration
Energy Type	Kundalini, raw earth energy

In the meditation position of choice; first ground and then do the Secret Smile.
Let your awareness drop down to your perineum. As you inhale feel the energy flow in through your perineum and up your spine. Watch the phosphenes behind your eyes as when you do this they tend to turn red.

2nd Chakra

The Second or Water Chakra is the center for our feelings and creativity.

Location	Abdomen, small intestine
Color	Orange
Key Word	Feeling, Creativity
Descriptors	Water elements and animals.
Source Of	Female power, feelings, creative energy, birth and gestation activity for babies, ideas, projects, etc.
Seat of	Female identity, awareness of feelings
Problems	Appendix disorders, kidney problems (childhood issues), issues from stored stuck or unexpressed emotions, PMS, ovarian disorders, creative blocks
Contains	Feelings of self and others
Physical Communication Style	Expressing feelings through the appropriate physical medium such as laughing, crying, screaming, etc.
Energy Type	Chi energy

In the meditation position of choice; first ground and then do the Secret Smile. Let your awareness drop down to the area about 2 inches below your beltline (the Hara or dan tien). As you inhale feel the energy flow in through your hara and up your spine. Watch the phosphenes behind your eyes as when you do this they tend to turn orange.

3rd Chakra

The Third or Fire Chakra is the power center and is where we store our judgments, opinions and beliefs about the world and ourselves.

Location	Solar Plexus
Color	Yellow
Key Word	Power
Descriptors	Air elements, birds
Source Of	Masculine power, intellectual understanding of the physical/worldly existence
Seat of	Male identity, self esteem, directed will
Problems	Digestive, metabolic disorders, weight problems
Contains	Opinions, Differentiated beliefs
Physical Communication Style	Intellectual understandings at the 'gut' level
Energy Type	Mental, intellectual

In the meditation position of choice; first ground and then do the Secret Smile. Let your awareness drop down to your Solar Plexus. As you inhale feel the energy flow in through your solar plexus and up your spine. Watch the phosphenes behind your eyes as when you do this they tend to turn yellow.

4th Chakra

The Heart or Wind Chakra is the melting pot for the divine energy coming down from the crown and the earth energy coming up from the root.

Location	Heart, sternum
Color	Green
Key Word	Love, healing
Descriptors	Earth elements, mammals
Source Of	Healing energy, dreams, innermost desires
Seat of	Compassion, relationships
Problems	Circulatory disorders, blood pressure problems, sleep disorders, relationship problems
Contains	The ability to relate
Physical Communication Style	Communicates physical/emotional needs through pain, heart pangs, tugs
Energy Type	Astral (connects to dream world and astral plane)

In the meditation position of choice; first ground and then do the Secret Smile.

Let your awareness drop down to your heart. As you inhale feel the energy flow in through your heart and up your spine. Watch the phosphenes behind your eyes as when you do this they tend to turn green.

5th Chakra

The Throat or 5th Chakra is our communication center. We express what we see, think, feel, desire and detest.

Location	Throat
Color	Blue
Key Word	Expression
Descriptors	Etheric elements, humanity
Source Of	Truth
Seat of	Wisdom, responsibility
Problems	Inability to say 'no' or 'yes', any disorders relating to the throat or mouth
Contains	The ability to define ourselves in the world
Physical Communication Style	Language, sounding, singing, toning
Energy Type	Etheric (emotional energy charged with spiritual awareness)

In the meditation position of choice; first ground and then do the Secret Smile.
Let your awareness drop down to your throat As you inhale feel the energy flow in through your throat and up your spine. Watch the phosphenes behind your eyes as when you do this they tend to turn blue.

6th Chakra

The "3rd Eye" or 6th Chakra is our inner/outer visual center.

Location	Forehead
Color	Purple
Key Word	Vision
Descriptors	Spiritualized humans, saints, spirits, gurus
Source Of	Insight
Seat of	Visions, visioning
Problems	Adolescent issues, eye problems, glandular problems, growth or development issues, problems planning for the future
Contains	Self image and means of shaping/correcting ones view of self and the world
Physical Communication Style	Uses ability to see, draw or project images to communicate
Energy Type	Cerebral (draws energy from the brain and 7th chakra)

In the meditation position of choice; first ground and then do the Secret Smile.
Let your awareness go to your third eye. As you inhale feel the energy flow in through your third eye and up through your crown

and out the top of your head. Watch the phosphenes behind your eyes as when you do this they tend to turn purple.

7th Chakra

The Crown or 7th Chakra is the "psychic center" for higher knowing and it receives the spiritual energies and guidance necessary to activate our purpose.

Location	Crown of the head
Color	White/clear
Key Word	Divinity
Descriptors	Spirits, God forms, angels, powers
Source Of	Divine awareness
Seat of	Our oneness with all
Problems	Cancers, bone disorders, schizophrenia, depression, ungrounded-ness, lack of direction
Contains	The receptive means for understanding our path and purpose
Physical Communication Style	Describes physical needs through our thoughts
Energy Type	Ketheric, a form of spiritual energy from beyond earths space/time

In the meditation position of choice; first ground and then do the Secret Smile. Let your awareness go to your crown chakra. As you inhale feel the energy flow in through your crown and back down to your heart. Watch the phosphenes behind your eyes as when you do this they tend to turn white.

Now start over and run the energy in through each chakra at a time in order. You can do this for as long as you like. I like to do it while driving on long trips.

Chapter 2

Other Chakras

You'll notice that I keep referring to the 7 *primary* chakras. We have other chakras in our palms and the soles of our feet as well as throughout our organs and the rest of our body. We even have chakras outside our body, below our feet and above our heads. You'll also notice that I didn't even get into the back side of the chakras in the chart above.

In all we have 32 chakras which all act in various ways and have various effects on our spiritual, physical, mental and emotional selves. A smart, curious person could spend a lot of time just researching all the various possibilities of the chakras and how they affect us.

I strongly advise anyone who wants a real understanding of themselves to devote some time to this.

Chakras balance each other

It's important to remember that the chakras balance each other. The Root chakra and the Crown chakra will both be affected when you work with either one of them, for instance, as will the 2nd chakra and the 3rd eye and so on.

As you begin doing the following exercises you'll see that working with the chakras can have a synergistic effect. As you begin cleansing and clearing the root chakra you'll also be activating the crown on a lesser level. When you follow this up with the chakra balancing exercises that I've put into the next chapters then you'll find that even though you're working with one certain chakra, the energy in all of the others is also affected.

Pay attention to what you see on the phosphenes behind your eyes as well as what you feel and experience emotionally. Your success when working with your chakras depends on your level of self awareness and your willingness to listen to and trust yourself.

As you balance, cleanse and open up your primary chakras you'll also, by extension, be opening up all the lesser chakras throughout your body. This process will continue *for the rest of your life*, so don't feel like you have to be in a hurry to get it done.

Warning!

It's imperative that you've developed the ability to have a positive outlook before you start working with the chakras. As you begin the cleansing process you're going to experience old, repressed emotions and memories. If you haven't learned to remain positive and release the energy then you can possibly get yourself into a lot of trouble here. This is where the support groups and internet discussion groups can really help. You are NOT alone with this stuff, no matter how it feels sometimes. ☺

Part 6

Chakra Exercises

Chapter 1

Drawing energy into the chakras

There are some very simple exercises that you can do for your chakras. As you get used to using the ones below you may discover variations and experiments that you can do with them also.

In the meditation chapters I went over how to 'draw energy' into yourself. This works very well as a chakra strengthening exercise.

In the meditation position of choice (even moving), go through the grounding and relaxation meditations. Begin the Drawing Energy meditation but rather than begin at the heart chakra begin at the Root or first chakra.

As you inhale draw the energy in through the chakra. Don't try to control the wheel or do anything with it, just let it spin as you energize it. Draw energy into it on the inhale and send energy back out of it on the exhale.

You may feel a variety of things with this exercise. You might feel the spinning of the chakras, or just a light area at the chakra as the energy flows in and out..

Continue this exercise up through the rest of the chakras.

Hugging the tree

Stand in the 'mountain' or 'standing stake' pose described earlier with your hands held about 8-12 inches out in front of your first chakra.

As you inhale feel the Earth energy rise up through your legs and fill your body, overflowing down your arms and out through your hands into the chakra. Let the energy continue to flow into the chakra as you exhale.

After a few minutes let your hands rise gently until they're in front of the second chakra. As you practice this you'll develop the ability to just feel when you should move your hands to the next chakra.

Continue this with each chakra. For the crown chakra hold your hands straight up at arms length above your head. Turn your palms inward and just let the energy flow.

Variations

You can do this using Earth energy as I just described. You can also use Universal energy and let it flow downward through your head until it fills your entire body and spills down your arms.

For the especially fun-loving you can combine this with the Yin/Yang meditation shown later in the book and combine both energies while visualizing the Yin/Yang symbol.

Releasing the old energies

Our chakras store memories and emotions as do our organs and muscles. Hopefully by now you've begun a steady yoga (or other moving meditative practice) and started cleaning some of that out manually. You should also be able to ground yourself properly and move your energy around.

As you pull energy into your chakras you'll occasionally come across memories or an emotion that's painful. In many cases it's good to take a moment and study the energy and see if there are any lessons to be learned from it, and then *just let it go*. Just release the energy and let it flow down into the earth like any other stress. If it seems to stick and develop a stress knot then find a good massage therapist, Reiki healer or acupuncturist (preferably all 3) to help manually release it.

You'll find that you have a tendency to laugh or cry much more easily. This is also one of the ways that the energy releases itself. I used to spend hours just driving through the mountains (and sometimes still do) just crying and laughing as this energy worked itself out. If you're married or involved with someone who isn't following the same path then it's imperative to have good lines of communication during this process also.

A special note for those in relationships

You're involved in a process that changes the way your energy flows, and the frequencies with which it flows. As your energy becomes stronger then the energy levels of your mate will also begin to increase, just by the constant contact with you.

What you do to yourself can easily affect those you're close to, so don't be surprised if your mate also begins to experience some clean outs. This can frequently happen after or during sex as this is all *sexual energy* and when you begin to crank it up then it can easily affect others.

Fortunately, I was aware of this fairly early on as I've had issues with several girlfriends who've experienced emotional cleanouts while having sex. If you're not really well attuned to your own process then it can be really disheartening when the object of your affections bursts into tears after making love. ☺

As usual communication is the key. You'll probably also begin to gravitate more towards sexual partners who are involved in metaphysics and energy work, or at least open to it. It can take a long time for a non-energy worker to get used to your energy and intensity.

If you're fortunate enough to be in a relationship with someone who can handle your energy then the practice of Tantra can open up some fun new areas of study. "The Big Red Book" can bring you and your partner hours of practice and exploration.

This is another area where the discussion groups can be extremely helpful.

Seeking help

It's entirely possible that you may stumble across a repressed emotion or memory that requires some professional help and counseling to cope with. If that happens then take your therapist a copy of this book in the hopes that it'll help them understand the process that you're involved with and why you're delving into these areas. It's important to remember that you are NOT alone with this process. There are some good resources available today in the form of support and discussion groups that can really help with your process. Take advantage of them and don't be afraid to get on and talk about what's going on with your practice. I can't tell you how many times someone has just made some offhand comment that unlocked doors for me.

I spent a decade completely alone, just stumbling through this. I see people today that just effortlessly flow through things that took me years to work out, simply because there are so many easily available resources now.

Dealing with Fear

"Pain is the mindkiller"
Myamoto Musashi

Learning to deal with your fears is a vital part of this process and not to be taken lightly. You'll see many warnings around the web and in various books about the Kundalini. As you can see from what I've written so far there are some *very real dangers* for the careless and un-aware.

In the early chapters of this book I addressed "Keeping a Positive Attitude" and "Having Faith". I can't stress the importance of these concepts enough at this point. When you break all your emotions down you'll see that they all stem from either LOVE or FEAR. On a moment to moment basis you have the ability to choose which of these you'll react from. Choose wisely.

Fear is much more than just the mindkiller. When you react from fear then you are reacting with a completely Id based response. It's one reason why I stress the necessity for a *good* martial arts regimen. Not to allow you to fight well, but to build your confidence and give you the ability to *keep from fighting and remain calm in desperate situations.*

Much of what you're learning in this book will stretch your comfort zones physically, mentally, emotionally and spiritually. Fools do indeed rush in where Angels fear to tread. At this point if you haven't developed the ability to calm your mind and your energy, as well as create a body and spirit that resonates with a loving, happy, compassionate energy, then you are setting yourself up for a trip through a paranoid, hellish, vitriolic existence.

To be afraid of your own energy is to be afraid of dealing with the most basic part of your *self.* To be afraid of another's energy is to fear the reflection of yourself.

Exercises like the *Secret Smile* and the *Inner Smile* can be a good defense against fear, as can good training and lots of practice. It's completely natural to get in over our heads and become afraid sometimes. When that happens then remember that there really is an infinite pool of loving, relaxed energy that you can tap into at any time.

I've also seen some otherwise excellent Chi Kung practitioners who caution against being "open" with your energy. Some of the reasons I've seen for this include the possibility of being attacked and also the fact that when your energy is open then you are "leaking" energy away from your body.

My usual response is "So what?" I'm not leaking it, I'm giving it away as it comes from a literally limitless pool. I don't have to hoard it or hide it. I'm so utterly unconcerned about being attacked that I won't even bother to address that, other than to point out that living in an armored existence also limits you.

There *are* times when it's good to pull your energy in and in effect disappear, but those applications are usually used in combat and intelligence gathering and aren't really useful here. Those applications are also NOT based in fear, but are purposeful.

There are dangers involved with energy work, just as there are dangers involved in any other facet of life. Training and self awareness is the way to deal with those dangers. The best thing that I can tell you here is that *love and compassion are the best armor that you can have.* Does that *always* work? Of course not, but neither does anything else.

Chapter 2

Basic Reiki

Reiki is an extremely useful tool for cleansing and balancing the chakras. I've used it for years and found innumerable benefits to it.

Basic Reiki

This is a very simplified primer on basic Reiki. It's intended as a basic lesson to help someone get started channeling the energy. Anyone interested in learning Reiki can download the Complete Reiki Course for FREE at www.robertmorgen.com/Reiki1.pdf

Clearing up some Reiki Myths

There are a few old myths and misunderstandings about Reiki that I'll take a moment to address.

The Attunement Process

One of the major myths in Reiki is that you must be attuned to Reiki by a 'master' to be able to use it. I've proven repeatedly in my own classes that this is NOT true and that the average person has the ability to use Reiki instantly.

The attunements make the connection to the energy stronger and cause a rapid cleansing of the body and the chakras, but this will happen gradually over time if you just keep using Reiki. Reiki is out there and available to everyone. You don't need anyone's permission or certificates to be able to use it to heal yourself, friends and family.

The Energy Exchange myth

A former Grandmaster of Reiki instituted the concept of energy exchange to validate charging extraordinarily high fees for master level attunements. Her position was that people wouldn't value something that was offered freely and I tend to agree with her.

However, if you remember the Law of Reciprocity that I mentioned at the beginning of the book, you'll also realize that merely by giving healing energy to another person you're making the world a better place. No exchange is necessary. You get back what you send out.

I have no qualms with a professional healer charging for services; just don't mislead anyone in the process.

What is Reiki?

Reiki is a Japanese phrase which means "Universal Energy". Its history is enshrouded in myth, legend and parable, but the simple fact is, it works. Reiki is simply the process of channeling Universal

Energy through oneself and into some one (or something) else. The vast range of uses for Reiki range from healing oneself to opening and balancing the Chakras and even charging objects and food with the energy.

Getting Started

Reiki is safe and simple to use. To get started simply sit or lie down in a comfortable position. Put on the music of your choice and relax. Place your hands over your face with your palms over your eyes. Touch your tongue to the roof of your mouth with the tip of your tongue just behind your front teeth.

As you inhale just open up and feel the energy flow down through the top of your head and down to your heart chakra, then feel it flow out along your arms and out through your hands and into your face. At the simplest level that's ALL you have to do. The energy will go wherever it's needed and do whatever is required of it. You don't have to send it anywhere in particular or try to control it.

Getting Deeper

Reiki flows through you simply by your *intent*. You just have to intend to open up to it and you'll find it readily available. You may feel many different things while giving yourself a Reiki treatment. Your hands or the part of your body covered by your hands may get hot, cold or tingly. Some people feel it very easily and others take awhile to open up to it. The simplest explanation that I've found is to think of what the emotion *Love* feels like, and then just relax and let it flow.

I always advise everyone to study Reiki. Any energy worker, massage therapist, healer, martial artist or metaphysician can greatly benefit from Reiki, and there are many FREE Reiki classes and sources of training available, as many of us try to make it as easily accessible as possible to anyone who wants it.

I hope this simple exercise helps some of you who've been interested in Reiki, but just haven't made the leap into studying it yet.

Chapter 3

Chakra Balancing

Here's a simple exercise that anyone can do using Reiki. It's simple and easy and you can do it even if you haven't been attuned to Reiki. It requires a basic knowledge of channeling Reiki energy, the positions of the 7 primary chakras and a willingness to spend some time making someone else feel good. Everything else is optional.

Setting the tone

I like to create a nice atmosphere when doing Reiki. I usually light up some nice incense and for music I usually use Nik Tyndall's *Reiki-Healing Hands* CD as it's also designed to help open the heart chakra.

Getting Started

Just lie down in a comfortable position and put a pillow under your knees to help take the strain off your lower back.

Place one hand over your crown and the other over your 1st chakra. Now just relax and open up to the energy and let it flow down through the top of your head, through your heart chakra and out through your hands. Spent several minutes here, or until you feel like it's time to change.

Next move one hand up to your 2nd Chakra and the other down to your third eye. Spend as much time as you need here, and then move one hand down to your Throat Chakra and the other up to your Solar Plexus Chakra. After you finish here then just switch your hands around to your chakras at random (including the Heart Chakra) and continue tuning them up for as long as you desire.

Getting Deeper

These exercises can obviously be enhanced by using the Reiki Symbols and by having the Attunements, but neither is really necessary. Over time your body will attune itself if you keep running the energy.

These exercises can also be enhanced by regularly practicing 'The 5 Tibetans' exercises, as they help tune and rejuvenate your chakras.

There are so many things that can be done, both with Reiki and your Chakra System, and the point of this exercise is to help you balance your energy and feel better. It's also about building up your own catalog of experience, as it's pretty hard for any teacher to tell you what a certain exercise should feel like when you do it. I can tell you how it feels to me when I do it, but it may feel differently to you when you do it yourself, so play with it and see how it feels.

This is also about learning to trust yourself and your own feelings and the only way to do that is play with your energy and have fun with it.

Chapter 4

Opening The Chakras

If you've been doing the exercises then by this point you should be in the process of opening and balancing your chakras in a very gentle and safe manner. The following exercises should be done *one chakra at a time* in the beginning. For the first few weeks do the chakras one per night. Do the Grounding and Secret Smile exercises first as you really want a happy, relaxed body for this. Give it a few weeks and then practice opening the first four, Root through Heart. Take your time with this.

Doing it this way helps *cool* the energy as you work up through the chakras. You *do not* want a blast of hot Kundalini rocketing up your spine into the base of your brain. You could go faster and get more dramatic results, but remember that everything balances between the dualities. The more dramatic your experience on one end of the scale the more dramatic the aftershock will be on the other polarity. The goal here is slow steady progress that doesn't turn your life upside down rather than a sudden eruption of Kundalini up your spine. The sudden eruption stories all sound cool when the survivor tells them years later at parties, but there's a long process in between, so take it slow and easy.

The simple secret to opening the chakras is the lotus flower. It has a root, a stem and the flower itself. Each Chakra also represents the flower and each chakra has a certain number of petals which correspond to the wavelength of the energy.

First chakra

After Grounding and the Secret Smile, just relax and let your senses fall down to your first chakra. Now visualize the first chakra as a red lotus flower with 4 petals. Allow the face of the flower to turn slowly and gently until it faces directly up your spine.

Allow the earth energy to flow through the four petalled lotus and gently up your spine, *changing colors as it goes through the other chakras and out through the top of your head*. Gently squeeze your sphincter and PC muscles on the inhale. On the exhale feel cool universal energy flow in through the top of your head and back down through your entire body.

Do this for about 20-30 minutes and then give yourself the Reiki energy balance as described earlier. Don't skip this step as it helps to equalize all your chakras to your growing energy levels.

Second Chakra

After Grounding and the Secret Smile, just relax and let your senses fall down to your second chakra. Now visualize the second chakra as an orange lotus flower with six petals. Allow the face of the flower to turn slowly and gently until it faces directly up your spine.

Allow the earth energy to flow through the six petalled lotus and gently up your spine, *changing colors as it goes through the other chakras and out through the top of your head.* Gently squeeze your sphincter and PC muscles on the inhale. On the exhale feel cool universal energy flow in through the top of your head and back down through your entire body.

Do this for about 20-30 minutes and then give yourself the Reiki energy balance as described earlier. Don't skip this step as it helps to equalize all your chakras to your growing energy levels.

Third Chakra

After Grounding and the Secret Smile, just relax and let your senses fall down to your third chakra. Now visualize the third chakra as a yellow lotus flower with ten petals. Allow the face of the flower to turn slowly and gently until it faces directly up your spine.

Allow the earth energy to flow through the ten petalled lotus and gently up your spine, *changing colors as it goes through the other chakras and out through the top of your head.* Gently squeeze your sphincter and PC muscles on the inhale. On the exhale feel cool universal energy flow in through the top of your head and back down through your entire body.

Do this for about 20-30 minutes and then give yourself the Reiki energy balance as described earlier. Don't skip this step as it helps to equalize all your chakras to your growing energy levels.

Fourth Chakra

After Grounding and the Secret Smile, just relax and let your senses go to your fourth chakra. Now visualize the fourth chakra as a green lotus flower with twelve petals. Allow the face of the flower to turn slowly and gently until it faces directly up your spine.

Allow the earth energy to flow through the twelve petalled lotus and gently up your spine, *changing colors as it goes through the other chakras and out through the top of your head.* Gently squeeze your sphincter and PC muscles on the inhale. On the exhale feel cool universal energy flow in through the top of your head and back down through your entire body.

Do this for about 20-30 minutes and then give yourself the Reiki energy balance as described earlier. Don't skip this step as it helps to equalize all your chakras to your growing energy levels.

Fifth Chakra

After Grounding and the Secret Smile, just relax and let your senses go to your fifth chakra. Now visualize the fifth chakra as a blue lotus flower with sixteen petals. Allow the face of the flower to turn slowly and gently until it faces directly up your spine.

Allow the earth energy to flow through the sixteen petalled lotus and gently up your spine, *changing colors as it goes through the other chakras and out through the top of your head.* Gently squeeze your sphincter and PC muscles on the inhale. On the exhale feel cool universal energy flow in through the top of your head and back down through your entire body.

Do this for about 20-30 minutes and then give yourself the Reiki energy balance as described earlier. Don't skip this step as it helps to equalize all your chakras to your growing energy levels.

Sixth Chakra

After Grounding and the Secret Smile, just relax and let your senses go to your sixth chakra. Now visualize the sixth chakra as an indigo lotus flower with two petals. Allow the face of the flower to turn slowly and gently until it faces directly up your spine.

Allow the earth energy to flow through the double petalled lotus and up through your crown and out to the universe. Gently squeeze your sphincter and PC muscles on the inhale. On the exhale feel cool universal energy flow in through the top of your head and back down through your entire body.

Do this for about 20-30 minutes and then give yourself the Reiki energy balance as described earlier. Don't skip this step as it helps to equalize all your chakras to your growing energy levels.

Seventh Chakra

After Grounding and the Secret Smile, just relax and let your senses go to your seventh chakra. Now visualize the seventh chakra as a violet lotus flower with a thousand petals. Allow the face of the flower to turn slowly and gently until it faces directly up your spine.

Allow the earth energy to flow through the thousand petalled lotus and up into the universe. Gently squeeze your sphincter and PC muscles on the inhale. On the exhale feel cool universal energy flow in through the top of your head and back down through your entire body.

Do this for about 20-30 minutes and then give yourself the Reiki energy balance as described earlier. Don't skip this step as it helps to equalize all your chakras to your growing energy levels.

The Lesser Kan and Li

After a few weeks of practicing one chakra at a time you can try the following exercise. By now you should be in the habit of Grounding and the Secret Smile. Remember the sphincter squeezes also.

First week
Practice drawing the energy up through the first two chakras. Visualize the lotus flower growing up out of the mud, firmly rooted, its orange six petalled face rising towards the sun. See the energy flow up through the orange lotus and change colors as it flows through the other chakras and out the crown and into the universe. Be sure to balance your chakras afterwards.

Second week
Practice drawing the energy up through the first three chakras. Visualize the lotus flower rowing up out of the mud, firmly rooted, with a stem holding its yellow ten petalled face, rising towards the sun. See the energy flow up through the yellow lotus and change colors as it flows through the other chakras and out the crown and into the universe.

Third week
Practice drawing the energy up through the first four chakras. Visualize the lotus flower rowing up out of the mud, firmly rooted, with a stem holding its green twelve petalled face, rising towards the sun. See the energy flow up through the green lotus and change colors as it flows through the other chakras and out the crown and into the universe.

By this point you should be developing the depth and experience to chart your own course with completing the energy. If the path isn't obvious by now then start over and take your time. Noone is on a schedule here and this is not something to rush into. At this point you'll probably go through a period of feeling very spiritually superior. Let it go to your head and then get over it.

Chapter 5

Damo's Cave

Damo's Cave is a form of an ancient Shamanic Journey in which the seeker travels internally. Damo is also known as the Bodhidharma or Daruma, depending on which version of the tales you read. Damo was the Hindu monk who traveled to China and taught the Shaolin Monks Kung Fu. It's a fun legend that may even be true. It's an interesting and fun exercise that can really teach you a lot about yourself. It's a great meditation for learning to visualize and fantasize, both of which are important skills for creating the world you want to live in.

This works better as a guided meditation as it allows you to concentrate on the imagery rather than trying to remember what comes next. You can either have someone read this to you or you can order the CD Set that accompanies this book.

Hit the position of choice and doing the Grounding and Secret Smile exercises. By now you should be able to do those pretty effortlessly. Feel your body becoming lighter and filled with relaxed, happy energy.

With your eyes closed and looking up into the third eye, see yourself floating in a calm sea. Try to make this as realistic as possible. Can you feel the warm water supporting you and smell the salt air?

In the distance is an island. You don't have to swim for it, all you have to do is relax and let the island come to you as you ride the ocean's currents toward it. As you get to the shore you can see the bright, sandy beach and a forest of palm trees up the side of a huge volcanic mountain. A trail leads from the beach up through the trees and up the side of the mountain.

As you walk across the sand you can feel yourself drawing energy from the ground up through your feet. You become stronger and more confident as you begin to walk up the trail through the trees.

Off to the left you can see the abandoned ruins of an old temple and a graveyard. There are also a couple of pools nearby. You go around these and continue up the trail. The climb becomes steeper and harder as you go and you feel yourself beginning to get tired. You lean against the trees and rocks and discover that you can also draw energy in through your hands, and this revitalizes you and gives you the strength to keep climbing.

Ahead of you the trail forks and you see that one fork leads around to a large cave. There's a guardian at the entrance of the cave who wears a long cloak and a cowl that masks its identity. You get closer to the cave and the guardian motions for you to enter. You can feel a strong sense of acceptance and the guardian bows to you, making you feel a bit like a king or a queen.

Inside the cave is a long, downward spiraling tunnel. The walls glow with a slight phosphorescence that allows you to see as you descend. The tunnel opens out into a large cavern with a faint glow of hot lava far back towards the rear. On your left is a podium upon which rests a large leather bound book. On the cover in gold letters is written "All Knowledge Is Power! Seeking Truth, First Look Ye Here."

Behind the podium is a room with a huge array of computers and electronics. There are three very comfortable looking captain's chairs in the room and a young man and woman working there. They don't see you yet.

To the right is a great stairway with five wide steps of different colors. At each step is a door.

The first step is red and the door is massive. You can see past it into a desert with a large stone city in the distance.

The second step is orange and the door is built like double Dutch doors. Beyond this door you can see a small stream that leads down to a huge lake or an ocean. In the distance is a ship coming in to the harbor.

The third step is yellow with an intricately carved door. Beyond is a city that's both ancient and modern and which shelters a wide variety of people, including some who look like elves. You can hear the faint tinkle of glassware and laughter if you listen.

The next step is green and opens out onto a bright blue, cloudless sky. You can see a bird floating gracefully on the updrafts outside.

The last step is tilted and spirals off into the distance fading through shades of violet and white. It seems to penetrate through the rock of the cave in the far distance.

In the center of the cave are your living quarters. You see a series of rooms that house your bedroom, bath, a personal dojo and instructor, stables, laboratory, machine shops, gear lockers, gardens, a library and a kitchen.

In one room you find a hidden doorway and in another is a trapdoor under the rug. You don't explore either at this time as they are both dark. In a room towards the back of the cave is an animal that seems to regard you as its master.

My cave was bare when I first got into it, but it's gradually taken on a very Oriental/Native American look as I've explored it and begun to furnish it more to my liking.

This is your space and you can do anything you like with it. Explore through the doors, interact with the people and animals. Open up the book and see what's in it. You'll find the gear lockers fully stocked with climbing gear, scuba gear, etc. As I've begun to trim down my possessions and build up my connections to the universal energy I've found that I need less gear for my explorations so I'm turning that space into a hydroponics greenhouse.

Get as real as you possibly can with this exercise. Try to smell the fragrances and feel the wind on your skin. Get as wild and crazy as you want to also. This is *your* space and anything goes.

Chapter 6

Travels in the Void

When you look up into your third eye and clear your mind completely you can enter a space that goes beyond the normal mundane world. The Void is a place completely outside of space and time where anything can, and often does, happen.

Eventually you'll run into something malignant while traveling in the void. You can look at these beings as anything you want. You can see them as spirits, demons, aliens, representatives of human evil, whatever. The important thing to remember at this point is that, while frightening, they don't have any corporeal form.

You are more powerful than anything you'll run into in the Void. Some of these critters feed off of fear, so when you give it to them they like it and they'll come back for more. You can avoid most of the beasties in the Void simply by not showing fear. Occasionally one may decide to test you and when that happens there are a couple of different strategies you can use.

Medicine shields and spears

If you go for the Native American style you can easily make a Medicine Shield and a Medicine Spear. These don't have to be full-sized as they are just symbolic. Make a hoop using a green sapling or tree branch, attach a piece of rawhide, buckskin, rabbit hide, etc. and then paint it with your own personal symbols. You can consecrate it if you desire by smudging it with a bit of sage and some sweetgrass and then offering it for service to whatever directions or deities appeal to you. Hang it on the wall.

A Medicine Spear can be as simple as a stick that you consecrate and use to symbolize a spear. Hang it with the shield.

When you're in the void and something wants a taste you can just summon these and they'll appear in your hands. I don't advise carrying them with you as it strikes a very defensive posture.

Armor of Light

Another defensive tactic is to just see yourself armored in strong bright light. Once again this can just be summoned, so you don't have to go around feeling like you're on the defensive.

Just eat it

If you don't want to bother with either of those then you can just swallow the beast, literally. It's only energy so just inhale it and get on with your trip.

These tactics all sound pretty weird, especially if you've never been in the Void, but really they're just confidence builders. If you have enough confidence then you really don't have to worry about using them. If something bothers you and you have the confidence then you can just wave it away and it'll go. I only included this section because people occasionally ask about what to do if they are attacked.

Part 7

Awakening

Chapter 1

Becoming your True Self

Awakening the Kundalini is actually a fairly simple process. People do it all the time without even meaning to, just in the course of their lives. The hard part of awakening doesn't have anything to do with connecting the energy; it's about living with the person who has awakened the energy and BE-ing that person.

Many people experience dramatic changes in their personalities and lifestyles after a Kundalini Awakening. Sometimes this is caused by the changes that come from cleansing and balancing the chakras. As all the accumulated stresses and memories dissipate and are dealt with the seeker finds that things that used to be earthshakingly important just don't matter anymore.

The brain and nervous system actually goes through a rewiring process as the body becomes used to running higher energies. Frequently the person in the midst of this rewiring process will experience shudders, called *kriyas*, which run through their muscles.

During this process the seeker often begins to see their life and their purpose here much differently. This, combined with the process of letting go of attachments and dropping the ego-based masks that we're all taught to wear can cause some pretty radical changes in a person's behavior.

On the other hand some people just hit the Kundalini like a speed bump and don't seem to make the same extreme changes to their life. Sometimes the answer is simply that they were already living their intended life and the dramatic changes just weren't necessary.

One reason that I stress the positive attitude and doing exercises like the Secret Smile is because this can be a pretty rough time, especially for those who tend to be negatively oriented. Don't be afraid to get onto the discussion groups and talk about this either. Most likely there will be someone else on there that's going through the same thing but doesn't recognize it.

Chapter 2

"BE" in the moment

One of the interesting aspects of Kundalini Awakening is its inherent chicken/egg quality. Did our lives change *because* our Kundalini awakened or did our Kundalini awaken because *we* changed our lives?

Many people pursue meditation, healing, martial arts and other pathways to personal mastery because they sense the need for change in themselves. They know that they need to become more, so they begin the process of *becoming*.

However, the thing I see from so many people is the expectation that something will happen suddenly and they'll immediately just *be* the person they want to be. That seems to be one of the misleading expectations about Kundalini Awakening; that they'll have this amazing experience and then just suddenly be enlightened.

For the most part it just doesn't work that way, unfortunately. I remember making the comment to Dr. Glenn Morris when I first met him that "rather than becoming

Enlightened, the Kundalini Awakening makes me aware on a moment to moment basis just how *Un*-enlightened I really am". Such a simple lesson that took so long to sink in.

This moment, right now, is the only one that really exists. The last moment has faded into some abstract, subjective past that only exists in our individual memories, and the next moment is part of a future that may never arrive. This breath, right now, is the only real breath, as the last one is gone and the next one isn't guaranteed. I once spent several minutes face down in the ocean, paralyzed and unable to move. Each time a wave hit me and turned my face up out of the water I took as big a breath as I could get and then held it, wondering if I was ever going to get another. Some of us need harsher lessons than others apparently. ☺

So the question becomes "What am I doing *right now*?" "Am I living the way I want to live *right now*, and if not then what can I do to make that happen?"

Most of us have at least a vague idea of who we think we want to be when we awaken to our true selves. Here's your Wake Up Call then. Start BE-ing that person *right now*! If you want to be like a Buddha then BE like a Buddha. If you see enlightenment as being nicer to others and treating them the way you want to be treated and loving them as you love yourself then do it, *right now*.

Chapter 3

Balancing the dualities

I feel that many of our issues with duality go back to our very basic nature, not our good/bad, male/female or light/dark side, but even deeper to the Id and Super-Ego. It's extremely easy to see these as the basis for all of the others with the battle being between the untrained, instinctive Id and the overly intellectual Super-Ego and the need for balance.

I wouldn't be surprised to learn that all of this started with some old shaman sitting around the campfire trying to put it into terms that his people could understand.

"Look at it this way" he might have told them, "On this side you have Order and Law and Creation, let's call that side God, and over here you have chaos and disorder and acting intuitively on your baser instincts, let's call that side Satan..."

Balancing the Masculine/Feminine

The Battle of the Sexes has raged for hundreds of years now and in my opinion it's really beginning to screw up the planet. We all have a masculine and a feminine side, and apparently most of us are severely unbalanced towards one or the other.

Some of the heinous acts of our major religions are designed to keep the feminine energies in check. Kundalini is by definition, sexual energy. Everything that lives is created through a sexual act of some sort and it's that very energy that we seek to elevate and awaken. Pick almost any major religion or path and you'll see some sort of sexual dysfunction displayed as celibacy, clitorectomies, or the domination of men or women.

What you're actually seeing here in many cases is the level of individual discomfort with their own internal energies, a non-acceptance of that part of themselves manifested in some sort of external sexual inequity. I won't argue that there are times when abstinence can be used to strengthen a spiritual journey, just like any other form of fasting. I will point out though that it's also frequently used as an escape that can leave the practitioner in a severely unbalanced state. Having occasionally experienced periods of abstinence for a variety of reasons (primarily by using my personality as a means of birth control) I can definitely say that it leaves one unbalanced and reactionary.

I believe the human body was intended to operate with a certain balance of male/female energies and that these energies are meant to balance one another just as in any of the other dualities. I also believe that it's possible to draw these energies from the world around us without the need for an actual sexual partner; I'm just not very good at it.

"The Big Red Book" officially known as *Sexual Secrets* (Douglas and Slinger) goes into a lot of detail on the various sexual energies and it's a lot of fun to read also. As with some of Mantak Chia's books on sexual techniques I can't recommend it strongly enough. I think the world would probably be a much better place if it were issued to everyone and we were tested on it regularly.

Balancing the Light and Dark

Integrating my dark side was a fairly torturous process for me, partly because I made it harder than it had to be. Apparently I do that a lot. ☺

One of the problems at the time was my inability to get out of my own way and I continually tried to micro-manage the process rather than giving in to it and going where it wanted to take me. Part of that was from my own misconceptions about the light and dark and my reactions to them.

Many of us spend a long time trying to suppress the various elements of our light and dark sides partially because we're taught to believe that light is *good* and dark is *evil*, as if the 2 extremes didn't exist in all of us.

For example, a lot of healers tend to shy away from their dark side. When it does manifest it's usually in some context that the healer may be shocked by or ashamed of. Thereafter the healer may have a negative connotation with the dark side of their being. Sometimes these connotations can come from events that happen when we're small children or even possibly be hold-overs from past lives.

It's important to find examples of the dark and light that can be manifested positively and enjoyably as everything has to balance. It's unnatural for us to always be one or the other. Music, dance, theatre, movies, martial arts and sexuality are some of the ways that you can find positive examples of both the dark and the light. In reality you can find positive examples anywhere, these are some that I personally enjoy.

This is where the self awareness part of Kundalini Awakening comes in. You have to know yourself well enough to become comfortable with all the aspects of your personality, and to find creative ways to balance your proclivities. If you spend all day giving Reiki treatments and listening to soothing new age music then take some time in the evening and pop in a suitably dark movie or some nice dark music on the stereo. If you choose the music then turn off the lights, close your eyes and do some moving meditation and ecstatic dancing. You might be surprised at what you're able to clean out of your system this way.

What's important here is to learn to be comfortable with your dualities, and then get beyond them. This can be a journey of self discovery that can take you places that you didn't know you could go.

Dealing with Negativity

Once you start to become comfortable with your dualities you can begin to associate with the positive (good for you) light and dark traits and abilities.

Keeping a positive mindset is extremely important here as you're pushing your comfort levels to new extremes. We usually lump negativity into the 'Dark' category, but having a negative attitude isn't a positive dark trait. ☺

Remember that this is all about developing your own personal mastery. When you give in to negative feelings and emotions then you are giving away your personal power.

Yin/Yang Exercise

Here's an exercise that I've been playing with for awhile now. I won't say that I *invented* it because when it comes to meditation there really is nothing new. It's all been done before. I can say however, that I didn't learn this from any external source, it's just something that came to me.

Pick the meditation position that you prefer and take a moment to ground yourself. You do this by letting your energetic roots grow down into the earth and feel the earth energy flow up into you on the inhale, all the way up over your head.

As you exhale release all your stress and tension and let it flow back down into the earth to be recycled. Feel your muscles relax as this stress bleeds out of your body and feel your connection to the earth increase as you draw in each breath. Do this as long as necessary to become relaxed and feel a good connection to the energy.

Now as you inhale, feel the dark earth energy flow up the back side of your body, while simultaneously opening up and feeling the light universal energy flow down through the crown of your head and down the front of your body.

As you exhale see the 2 bands of energy swirl through you and into a yin/yang symbol that encompasses you. Continue at this level til you can do that with one breath comfortably.

The next step is to let loose of your perceptions and *become* the yin/yang symbol. Feel yourself expand beyond your usual physical boundaries with the light and dark energies swirling through you in perfect balance. If the energy wants to continue spiraling then let it.

Now begin to expand yourself, feeling the connectivity to the light/dark energy in everything around you. It's all the same energy and the parts of it that are in you are also the parts of you that are in it. Feel your energy expand til it fills (feels) the room, now let it expand to fill your house, your city, your state. Continue expanding out through the solar system, then the universe.

This is the energy that's all around us all the time. We're as much a part of it as it's a part of us, and in reality there's *no difference* between it and us. We/it encompass everything and we're/it's the basic building blocks for everything that ever was or is.

It's the proper balance of the light/dark, masculine/feminine, good/bad and positive/negative that holds everything together. "For every action there's an equal and opposite reaction" is not just a good idea, it's the law.

Take some time here and feel the connections to the universe within and without. *Feel* the swirl of the galaxies within you and visualize them as tiny yin/yangs all swirling together inside a larger yin/yang which is also just another swirl and realize (make REAL) that the dualities don't really exist, that they are just perceptions of the same reality.

Now choose one of the swirling yin/yangs at random and let yourself fall into it. This should be easy since (sense?) your connection to everything also gives you unlimited abilities. As you fall into this swirling galaxy you can see that it's made up of billions of swirling little solar systems all made up of little yin/yangs. Choose one at random and flow into it. See the little yin/yangs rotating around a larger one in the center. Choose one of these at random and flow down to it. When you look more closely at it you can see that it is also made up of billions of swirling, individual yin/yangs. Choose one of these and flow into it.

Now without letting go of your connection to the universe, can you open your eyes and feel the light/dark energies swirling all around you? Did you come back down to the same room and body and mindset that you left? Does it matter?

Play with this as there are infinite possibilities and energies to explore.

Chapter 4

Dealing with the ego

We spend a lot of time dealing with self awareness and self consciousness and self esteem, so who exactly is this *self* and why does it matter?

Webster's defines the *Ego* as "the self, especially as contrasted with another self or the world"

The *Super-ego* is defined as "one of the three divisions of the psyche in psychoanalytic theory that is only partly conscious, represents internalization of parental conscience and the rules of society, and functions to reward and punish through a system of moral attitudes, conscience, and a sense of guilt"

The *Id* is defined as "one of the three divisions of the psyche in psychoanalytic theory that is completely unconscious and is the source of psychic energy derived from instinctual needs and drives"

Great, just when I was feeling better, now I discover that I've got a divided consciousness. So what does it all mean exactly?

When Webster's mentions "the three divisions of the psyche in psychoanalytic theory" what they are talking about is the Conscious self or Super-ego, and the Subconscious self or Id, and the Ego, which is a combination of both. So in short, our ego is that which defines us and separates us from all the other egos out there and provides us with the framework for our reactions and responses to external and internal stimuli. It's both who we've learned to be and who we always were combined into who we *think* we are now.

One of the challenges that many of us face is learning to release the programming in our super-ego and let the natural expression of our id have more control. We seek to access more of our subconscious abilities and break free of the restraints that tie us down, to bypass the mental/emotional boundaries and experience the oneness of the universe and everything in it...you get the picture.

One of the problems that many of us have is that we are programmed from birth to *believe* various things, depending on the culture we grew up in. I grew up in a staunch Methodist community that firmly believed in an omniscient God and the miracles of the Bible while simultaneously scoffing at the metaphysical and supernatural. I learned early NOT to point out the similarities and when I was older I went through a fairly lengthy process of deciding which parts of the programming were useful and which could be discarded. Religion is just the easiest example, but there are many others.

We spend our lives learning how to be the people we become. We learn various *mores* and *norms* according to the society we live in. Since most of us are already outside what's 'normal' for our societies then I probably don't have to spend much time with this.

Some of this programming is useful and it lets us move through and function within our society. Some of it is useless and exists merely to keep us in line with whichever religious, economic, political, social order that happens to dominate at the moment. Some of it is destructive and designed specifically to prevent you from accessing your subconscious energies, preventing you from really thinking on your own and developing your Self in the directions that *you* think it should go.

In contrast the Id (or maybe just my Id) tends to be untrained to function in society and has very little worry about what's 'normal' or even polite. It's like a big, tough 6 year old kid. Just because something is an instinctive reaction doesn't necessarily mean that it's correct within the social context. When I see someone abuse an animal or a child my first response is to do to *them* whatever they are doing to the victim. I'm very Old Testament that way sometimes, but is that the correct response according to the laws we live under? Is it the correct response according to the laws of compassion and reciprocity? Sometimes a thoughtful solution can be better for everyone.

Rising above the Id is just as important as overcoming the Super-ego. Many of us have very unbalanced responses that are based in the Id rather than the Super-ego. Did you ever meet someone who tended to be very paranoid and reacted with violence as a first solution? In many cases the 'warrior' mentality is very Id based, as is the 'nurturer' and the 'shaman'.

The Super-ego and the Id

So what is the correct balance? The challenge here is to develop enough internal and external awareness to be able to go through and keep or discard the programming as we see fit. We have to go through and thoughtfully, purposefully think about what's important and how we should react to the various stimuli that bombard us constantly.

There are a few guidelines that you can go by that will help the process. Most religions are liberally sprinkled with these and if you apply them then they'll help act as a filter between the Id and Superego. I've seen about 20 different translations of "Do unto others as you'd have them do unto you", for instance. Personally I try to keep in mind that there are only two ways to respond to any given moment, through LOVE or through FEAR. On a moment by moment basis I always try to be aware of my responses and see which of those is dominant. Hopefully some day I'll be good at it.

The Super-ego and the Id will always be the defining factors of your ego, but fortunately your Ego is also the defining factor of the Super-ego and the Id. Through study and meditation you begin the process of shaping the Id and Super-ego and therefore the Ego, creating a single balanced entity, much like the Yin/Yang.

Chapter 5

Dropping our Masks

In a sense it's like we're each wearing a mask. We each have a set of pre-programmed responses to just about any external/internal stimuli and it's these programmed responses that make it so easy to occasionally bend and twist entire societies. These masks are the external personalities that we show others, and believe it or not, other people rarely see us as we see ourselves.

Beyond that, the masks we wear are also programmed with our memories and likes/dislikes at a personal level. They're an amalgam of everything we've done, both good and bad, as well as our views of ourselves. It's also possible to have an entire series of masks that you wear at different times and places. Do you act differently around certain people, or in certain places? Are those actions the result of self-awareness on your part or simply pre-programmed responses that you do automatically?

One of the things that happens with the Kundalini is that all the masks are stripped away. Suddenly you're left with a completely blank slate and it's up to you to decide what should be there. It's one of the reasons why some people have such radical changes to their personality after the Kundalini.

A lot of people also hide behind their masks and it can be extremely frightening when those masks no longer hide them from themselves. It's one of the reasons I'm constantly prattling on about intention and awareness and having a positive attitude.

The good news is that you don't have to experience a Kundalini Awakening to begin the process of dropping the masks. As you get deeper into the self-awareness process you'll begin to question some of the things you do and the reasons you do them. As you expand your awareness you'll be able to have different views of your own actions as well.

The simplest way to begin stripping these masks away is to look at your responses to external/internal stimuli. Do you respond primarily from the Super-ego (conscious) or the Id (subconscious) parts of your ego? How's that working out for you? Are there times when you'd like to respond more consciously and other times when you feel like your intellect gets in the way?

As you journey through your own self-awareness you'll find that you can begin changing your responses, and therefore changing your masks.

Part 8

Personal Mastery

Chapter 1

Dealing with anger

"When you are offended at any man's fault, turn to yourself and study your own failings. Then you will forget your anger."
Epictetus

As humans we have to deal with anger on a fairly constant basis. Some of us tend to be a little quicker to anger than others, but in general anger is one of the daily trials that we all have to work towards overcoming.

Dealing with anger brings us to some of the core principles of Kundalini Awakening, namely awareness. It's very easy to become stressed and then lose our tempers. It's incredibly hard at first to deal with some of the unfairness of life without getting angry and upset, but that's exactly what you have to learn to do. This was (and still is) a very long journey for me and I'm still being tested fairly regularly with no reason to believe that the tests will ever stop.

For example I was recently filling out my financial aid paperwork to go back to college and take some classes. In the process I discovered that the IRS had apparently lost *every one* of my tax returns since 1999. Only a few months ago this would have sent me into a rage (and a righteous one too!) yet this time I tried to remember that I was supposed to be handling this properly. During the entire ordeal (about 20 hours worth of phone calls, wrong instructions and outright ineptitude from the bureaucracy), I tried to remember to make things as pleasant as possible for the person on the *other end* of the conversation. While I probably could have handled it better, I still showed a marked improvement over how things would have been even a few years ago.

Like any other real change in our lives, dealing with anger is an incremental process. It's all about winning the little victory right now rather than worrying about winning the war on anger. As humans we'll probably never eradicate anger, but we can develop better strategies for dealing with it.

Identifying the causes

Here are a couple of examples of things that make me angry. We all have a list like this, and my advice here is to actually write it out and then write out the solutions for it.

Cause #1 - I've found that I'm most likely to get angry when I feel like I'm running late or short of time.

Solution – If it turns out that I'm running out of time, for whatever reason, I try to call ahead and make other arrangements for my appointments. While this necessity can still make me unhappy, it's at least a positive step and keeps me from being any ruder than I can help to the people waiting on me.

Cause #2 – I have a very low Stupidity Tolerance. I find incompetence and ineptitude to be one of the most amazingly rude things imaginable and a symbol of a business owner's lack of respect for their customers.

Solution – Lighten up, Old Man! We've all been new on the job or thrown out to the wolves without proper training. Take a minute and try to view things from the stupid-ees point of view and it may turn out that the situation isn't really anyone's 'fault'. Try to see the humor in it and see if it can all be turned into a joke.

Another tactic that I use in general and that I have pretty good results with is to view *everything* as a test. This works well for my personality type and may not work at all for others, but give this a try and see. Try the 'Sacred Space' test and let me know how it works for you.

To do the "Sacred Space' test first you have to understand that you can't change the world, but you can change the area directly around you, your bubble of influence.

With that in mind the test is to always have a bubble of happy sacred space around you, no matter what's going on. As your awareness increases you may find this easier to do. You are a living, breathing sacred space generator and everyone who comes in contact with you enters your area of sacred space and therefore should pass out the other side of it feeling better than when they went in to it.

The challenge with this is to feel that way about everyone, no matter how they've treated you, or how stupid, rude inept or downright mean they act. We all have the ability to be total jerks. Just as we've accidentally shown our bad sides to others, then others will show their bad sides to us. It's entirely possible that the one bad moment you witness from your adversary may be the only bad moment that person has ever shown. Judging them as a perpetual jerk may be as utterly unfair as the times when others judged you as a perpetual asshole.

When you bring the jerk into your bubble of sacred space then your goal at that point is to make *their* day better. Get beyond your own ego and the attitudes of "How dare they treat ME that way" and see if you can help break them out of their bad mood. Look at it like a game. Have fun with it.

Does this always work? Of course not. Sometimes the other person is still going to be a jerk, and sometimes in the case of a potentially violent situation this tactic may still not be enough to avoid the confrontation. As I often point out in my martial arts classes "You may still find it necessary to bend, fold and spindle an attacker, but at least this method keeps you from doing it in anger or hatred".

Another thing to remember about anger is that the usual response to it is more anger. What's the first thing that you feel when someone becomes angry with you? If you're like most of us then you also begin to get angry. It develops into a circle and keeps growing until it either spills over or sanity prevails.

The thing to remember with anger is that it's just like love. Someone can give you all of it that they want to, but it's up to you to *accept* it. Like the old example the monks use; if someone offers you a cup of tea and you refuse it then whose tea is it? It still belongs to them. If someone offers you anger and you refuse it then whose anger is it?

The next time you feel yourself becoming angry try this:

Begin your belly breathing drawing your breath deep into your hara. Let your muscles relax and let any tension flow out and down into the earth. As you inhale feel the earth energy flow up into you until it fills your entire body. On your exhales continue to let stress and tension flow out.

Begin drawing chi in through your liver. Don't worry if you don't know where your liver is, just open up and intend for the energy to flow into it and you'll eventually be able to actually feel your liver as you do this. Experiment and play with this. If your concentration is good then if nothing else it may take your mind off whatever you're angry about.

Remember that the Law of Reciprocity applies here also so if you send out anger then you'll receive anger in return.

Forgiveness

Of course, since none of us are perfect it's important to remember about forgiveness. When someone ticks you off the first thing to remember once you cool down is to forgive them for whatever they did to make you angry. This is extremely important because until you do this then you're still carrying the seeds of that anger around with you. Take a moment to forgive them for whatever moronic, utterly imbecilic action they committed, and then forget about it.

Of course, you also have to remember to forgive yourself. Most of us get just as annoyed with ourselves for losing control and giving in to the anger as we do at the person who inspired it. This is just one more area where keeping a positive attitude can be helpful.

Take a moment to critique the incident without assigning blame to either party. Look at the lessons learned and see what you could have done better and then forgive everyone involved and get on with your life.

Righteous anger

Of course, looking at the world today it makes you think that there are times when we *should* be angry. Human Rights abuses, starvation, injustice, etc. When you start getting mad about those things where do you stop? It might sound perfectly reasonable if you say "I'm only going to be righteously angry about the worst injustices and then stamp them out". If you're amazingly effective (more so than anyone has ever been) then you'll single handedly make the world a better place. However, you'll reach a point where you've cleaned up the entire planet and you begin to vent your righteous anger on some guy who spits on the sidewalk because that's the worst thing that's left.

Of course no matter how angry you get you can never stamp out injustice or abuse. Those things are part of our basic nature and you can't be angry about our basic nature, you can only accept it. Once you accept it then you can get beyond it.

Even righteous anger is subject to the Law of Reciprocity also. You may feel justified at being angry at the person who screwed up, but we all screw up occasionally. Personally I'd prefer to give compassion rather than anger (and I eventually hope to get good at it). When you react out of compassion then at least you don't have to worry about anger degenerating into hate.

Chapter 2

Using Compassion in everyday life

Compassion is simply the way we feel towards others. At any given moment we have 2 ways to respond to whatever happens. We can respond through fear, or we can respond through love. It's exactly that simple. The goal is to develop our own awareness to the point that we can always decide in an instant which way we want to respond.

This tends to be one of the areas that I have to constantly struggle with. I try to remember on a moment to moment basis that it should be a pleasure for another person to interact with me because I *should* always be relating to them from a loving and compassionate viewpoint. Of course this is the point where the little devil on my shoulder points out that the *best thing for some people* is a good swift kick in the ass.

So how do you temper compassion and mercy with reality? In my martial art classes I always teach the non-lethal, non-damaging techniques first. The point is not to hurt the person who attacks you, for instance, but merely to redirect them and get the point across to them that you're someone who shouldn't be attacked in the first place. Of course if you get to the point of physical violence then odds are that you've screwed up at the other levels.

My buddy Jeff is a street cop for a small town police department in Northeastern Colorado. He's in one of the professions where use of force is occasionally necessary. One of the ways that he's experimented with using compassion on the job is to open up his heart chakra and send green, compassionate energy to the people he deals with. He told me that when he started doing that it dramatically reduced the chances that a confrontation would escalate into violence. I've used similar techniques before when dealing with people in customer service and found that the anxiety level drops noticeably.

The next time you're in a 'discussion' with someone who wants to be argumentative try this;

Slow your breathing and remember to breath down into your hara. Relax your muscles and let all the tension drain out, then allow the grounding earth energy to flow up from your feet and let your entire body fill up with it, letting it overflow down into your arms and hands.

Keep your mind as clear as possible, send your awareness down to your heart chakra and draw energy into it. Feel it relax and expand as it energizes and then let your awareness expand outwards carrying with it a solid green wave of compassion. You can visualize this by seeing a bright green bar of light extend out from your chest to the chest of the person you're talking to. If you want you can let that green light expand until you are both inside a huge circle of compassion.

Experiment with this. You can also play with other colors and try various colors in different situations. As with anything else the more you use it the better you'll be at it.

Chapter 3

Spiritual Integration

"Soul development should take precedence over all things."
    Edgar Cayce

Are we spiritual beings having an earthly experience or are we earthly beings having a spiritual experience? Who said we have to be one or the other? Are the two mutually exclusive?

The thing that's been most interesting to me about the entire Kundalini process is the fact that I'm so much closer to my true spiritual self now than ever before. It's astounding to me to be able to feel past my physical body and connect to something larger and more ancient. As usual this is part of a larger process and it's one that's continually ongoing as I learn more and loosen up more.

Developing our spirituality is what it's about for most of us, although for a long time I never thought about exactly what that means. If we look at the overall picture and get beyond the shortness of lifespan for our physical beings we can see the longevity of our spirit. I like the idea that we come back over and over and learn lessons at the soul level. From that perspective the life we live has far reaching consequences for the hard headed as I can think of several parts of this life I wouldn't want to have to repeat just to get the proper remedial training.

The process of integrating yourself spiritually, mentally and physically can be a very long process. It requires a lot of self awareness and it's probably a somewhat different process for everybody. As usual many of us in Western society are at a disadvantage because we expect to see instant results.

There isn't much that I can tell you beyond that as you'll have to just put the time into it and do the work.

Chapter 4

Living With Abundance

"Every person, all the events of your life, are there
because you have drawn them there.
What you choose to do with them is up to you."
Illusions, Richard Bach, Delacorte Press, New York,
1977

"Poverty is God's way of saying 'you're a failure'"
Anonymous (an ancient Greek philosopher) ☺

The natural attitude of the awakened,
balanced, sentient being is one of abundance
and plenty. When you have the ability to
connect to the universe at it's core and
actually become one with it then there just
isn't room for the attitudes of deprivation or
poverty. The universe isn't deprived or
impoverished. It's huge; it's full of fantastic,
wondrous, amazing creations that we as
humans aren't big enough to understand.
We as spiritual beings, however, have the
ability to interact with it and connect to it
and take part in it.

For the seeker who lives with constant
self-awareness, deprivation and lack are
symptoms of imbalance. That's not to say
that those who suffer poverty are
unenlightened, just that some forms of
poverty are symptoms of imbalance.

I should clarify a few things at this point. If you *want* to be a monk and shave your head and be celibate and not own anything then that's a choice, and terms like lack and poverty don't apply. If you decide to get rid of everything you own and just live free of the attachments and wander the Earth as a spiritual being in human form then that's also a choice.

When I talk about poverty I mean the impoverished *mindset*, rather than the lack of stuff or money. It's this impoverished mindset, rather than the lack of money, that makes people poor and keeps them there.

Another good point is that often people may have some hold-over from a past life, such as a vow of poverty that they still live up to. That's where your self-awareness comes in and allows you to get past it and then begin living the life of abundance.

When I was a kid growing up in the foothills of North Carolina we hardly ever had money. We usually raised a garden and kept animals for the freezer. In the summer mom would can up the vegetables from the garden so we'd have something for the winter. While my parents would worry about money, they always made sure that my sister and I had shoes and decent clothes to wear to school. It never occurred to us that we didn't live in a time of abundance. Even when times were hard we had everything we needed. The times when we felt a *lack* of money were times when we wanted some external luxury. Of course growing up the way I did also 'programmed' some attitudes into me. The section that comes next is a posting I made on the Kundalini Awakening Discussion Group about that and the process that I was going through at the time.

Kundalini lessons about money

I've been going through an interesting growth period lately that I thought I'd share, as some of the lessons were pretty profound (at least for me).

I've written before about my Awakening and the joys and tribulations since, and I've also mentioned that it's an ongoing process which, as far as I can tell, doesn't really end til you shuffle off this mortal coil. Then you get to come back and start over.

The last couple of years or so have been a really interesting period, partly through the guidance and help from both Dr. Glenn Morris and Susan Carlson, and it's interesting how much progress I've made and how far I still have to go.

I've recently come to an interesting new period in my life, thanks mostly to my other half, Anya. Living with her (and my step-son Jake) has opened up new areas and forced me to deal with things that I was always able to avoid before. When you're a modern day gypsy bouncing around in an old RV it's really easy to have a casual attitude about living in our society, but settling down really brings on the new challenges. Most of what I'm learning now is probably old hat to those of you who've led stable, settled down lives, but it's a hell of an adventure for me, even at my age.

The primary things that I'm dealing with lately are financial. I've always been able to make money, but in the last few months I've come to realize that I've always had bad attitudes about it, and I see the same attitudes reflected over and over from the people around me. It was a big shock for me to realize how much my attitudes were actually limiting me. It was shocking because most of what I do is about rising above limitations and creating my own realities, and then realizing how badly I was doing in this other area.

Susan Carlson mentioned to me several times last year that I could learn a lot from Stuart Wilde's books, and I finally got around to reading *The Trick to Money is Having Some.* I have to admit that she was exactly right!

I followed that up with *Rich Dad, Poor Dad* and what I learned there was just as shocking, so in the hopes that some of you learn easier than I do I'll pass on some new revelations (apparently only new to me, but what the hell).

I grew up in the foothills of North Carolina as a poor country boy and most of the time money was a tool that we just didn't have. Our "reality" was that we had to struggle just to have *enough to survive.* While the concept of abundance was nothing new to us, we saw our abundance in what we could grow and make rather than what we could buy, and while those skills are definitely valuable, it's a very limiting attitude to have.

So within my 'reality' money wasn't really a tool that was very prominent in my toolbox, even though it was consistently one of the factors that prevented me from doing the things I needed to do.

Many of my attitudes came from the fact that I'm just not interested in money for its own sake. I'm pretty unimpressed by the people I've met who's primary characteristic seems to be that they have lots of money.

Also it's easy to develop bad attitudes when we see the evils done in the name of money, so for a long time my *reality* remained that I was working to have 'enough to survive'.

Another interesting factor is that many of us in western society are taught to believe that we don't *deserve* a lot of money. We're taught to *want* it, but not to *believe* that we deserve it, which only seems like a paradox til you think about how our consumer culture is driven by desire and want, rather than need.

What I finally realized is that I have to expand my reality and shake off the bad attitudes. Money is a fact of life in our modern world. It's a tool that too many of us are taught to ignore and misuse, and just because many of the world's ills and evils are conceived to get it doesn't mean that we should ignore the fact that many of the modern worlds *good* things are caused by it also. The fact that I can write this article and instantly send it out to hundreds of people all over the world is just one example.

I expect the next few months to be a very interesting and rewarding period as I learn more about this 'new' tool and how to effectively use it. Many of the healers and new agers that I know also have similar attitudes to those that I always had, so I thought I'd bring this up here.

I'm sure that many of you may have some interesting feedback.

The period since I wrote that posting has indeed been very interesting as I learn more about living with the attitude of abundance. If you haven't done so I strongly urge you to take the time to read Stuart Wilde's *The Trick to Money is Having Some* and Robert Kyosecki's *Rich Dad, Poor Dad.*

Chapter 5

Death and Reincarnation

"You're going to die a horrible death, remember. It's all
good training, and you'll enjoy it more if you keep the
facts in mind.
Take your dying with some seriousness, however.
Laughing on the way to your execution is not generally
understood by less advanced life forms, and they'll call
you crazy."
Illusions, Richard Bach

"I offer thanks to those before me,
that's all I've got to say.
Maybe you squandered big bucks in your lifetime,
and now I've got to pay.
Then again it feels like some sort of inspiration,
to let the next life off the hook.
She'll say 'Look what I had to overcome from my last
life; I think I'll write a book.'
How long til my soul gets it right?"
Galileo by the Indigo Girls

One of the perennial questions when it
comes to spirituality is "Where do we go
when we die?" All the major religions have
ways of dealing with this. In fact that's one of
the purposes of religion.

An interesting side effect that I've seen
in the handful of people I've met who've
actually awakened their Kundalini seems to

be a complete lack of fear concerning death as well as a firm belief in reincarnation. This isn't reincarnation in the sense that the exact same person that we are now will return to live again. It's more a recognition that the soul is immortal and that we come back here on a quest for further development on a larger level.

Of all the philosophies I've seen so far Tibetan Buddhism seems to make the most sense. The idea that we come back to achieve and learn certain things during our limited human lifetime is the only idea that's ever made sense to me intuitively.

Some of this is borne out through the study of the chakras and their ability to hold onto memories and contracts from past lives. There's a mounting pile of evidence from hypnotic past life regressions that's hard to ignore without some deeply ingrained programming that lets you argue against it. I find the usual "It's not true because God said so in the Bible" argument to be exceptionally weak to the point of becoming boring. Apparently a lot of things aren't mentioned in the Bible, which doesn't negate it as a historical and spiritual document and a lot of fun to read and debate.

The feeling that I've developed over the past few years, and it's just that, my feeling, is that we as a spiritual beings have certain things that we need to learn. We come here (Earth) over and over until we've finally learned enough to move on to whatever the next level of existence may be. It's kind of like an eternal cosmic video game where you have to keep going back to the beginning of each level and doing it over until you learn how to beat it. (Who said Nintendo was useless?)

My feeling is that before our re-birth we actually devise a plan and leave ourselves clues about where we're supposed to go and what we're supposed to learn. It makes perfect sense to me that this plan could also include who our parents are and the part of the world that we'll be born into as the lessons there can be extremely strong. At that point it's up to us to develop the awareness to follow the clues and learn to listen to our inner voices. It's as good a reason as any for why humans can feel so out of place and be looking for something 'more' from their lives.

I've occasionally talked to some of the Buddhists who seem to echo that theory almost exactly. I find that interesting since I'm not very devoted to any of the ism's.

In *Occult Tibet* J.H. Brennan points out that "According to Tibetan doctrines there are six possible "realms" into which you could be born, each one the result of your particular karmic trace. These are, in reverse order of comfort, the Hell Realm, the Hungry Ghost Realm, the Animal Realm, the Human Realm, the Demi-God Realm, and the God Realm".

As he points out, it's hard to tell whether the ancient Tibetans were referring to other planes of existence, or whether all the realms actually co-exist here on Earth. It's fun to debate it in either direction.

Contracts from past lives?

An especially interesting idea in chakra studies is that apparently we can carry over firmly held beliefs, both positive and negative, from past lives. In effect we're still honoring a contract that we made in a past life. In some cases the past programming is held in the chakras and causes the victim to continuously act out whatever the contract may have been.

Given the fact that the chakras can store information about every aspect of our lives it stands to reason that these contracts could be anything from a vow of poverty to a reluctance to eat green beans.

As you get deeper into your chakra studies and begin to learn more about your self then keep this in mind. There may be areas in your life that will require you to put some real effort into sorting out and it could be caused in part by these past life vows.

I think a lot of the attitudes about money can be attributed to past life vows of poverty. So many people in the metaphysical circles have bad attitudes about money and seem to be constantly working through it, just as I am.

Another interesting thought came up recently. Many of the folks who travel in the metaphysical circles today were probably healers, priests and shamans in past lives and still have the memories of the tribe taking care of them. Today the average healer or shaman has to have a day job and do their life's work after hours, yet they remember, at a soul level, the times when money and material possessions weren't necessary. Sometimes it's hard to break out of that.

With that in mind it's no surprise that many of us have problems in thinking positively about money. We especially seem to have problems anytime we're mixing money and spirituality. Often we feel that we shouldn't be charging money for anything related to our spiritual teachings and pathways.

At the same time, we no longer live in a world where the 'tribe' takes care of us, so it becomes necessary to have a way to defray expenses, especially when so many of us tend to travel to other cities and teach seminars and workshops.

Just something to think about.

Chapter 6

Becoming who we're supposed to be

Our place in the world

It's not unusual for humans to spend a lot of time wondering why we're *here* and where is *here* and what does it all mean? It's part of our natural curiosity of life but it's also part of a deeper drive to follow the plan we made for ourselves before our re-birth.

One of the great advantages with the Kundalini is that once the chakras begin the process of cleansing and balancing then it's possible to get a much clearer view of life's purpose.

In my personal experience, one of the important effects of my Kundalini Awakening was that I was finally able to figure out why I'm here and begin putting my life into some sort of perspective. A lot of people are fortunate in that they really don't have to deal with this. I've met people who seemed to always know exactly why they were here and what they were supposed to do with this lifetime in order to develop their souls for the next level.

My path was much different. I spent decades wandering around learning different skills and having a wide variety of experiences. For a long time I felt like I was on the outside of our society looking in, trying to figure out why I couldn't just settle down and get a good job and raise a family the way we're taught that we should. For over a decade after I experienced the first Kundalini I literally felt driven to go places and learn a strange group of skills. It was only after I met other people who'd also had Awakenings and began learning from them that I was able to open up my awareness and see the bigger picture.

As I look back on it now I can see that I was always doing exactly what I was supposed to be doing and that all of a sudden I've arrived at a point where I have enough grey hair to be taken seriously, enough experience to back it up and a unique skill-set to bring it all together and make it work. Once I figured out that I should just have a little faith and go where I'm supposed to go and do what I'm supposed to do, then all the stress and angst about my 'place in society' just went away and I was able to really make some progress internally.

As usual, *awareness* is the key to learning about our true selves. I stumbled around in the dark for a long time, driven by something that I was unaware of, but fortunate in the fact that I went where I was led nonetheless. My awareness was one of negativities though, as I couldn't see the possibilities, only the *im*-possibilities. For instance, I *knew* that I couldn't settle down and raise a family, but couldn't understand why. I knew that I wanted to go to college and learn, but couldn't see the point to pursuing the usual career paths.

Once I began to expand my awareness (starting with the breath, like usual) then I was able to begin to see a larger picture and have it make sense. It's a little like standing too close to a painting. It's out of focus and just a jumble of colors, but as you move back slightly and expand your awareness the colors transform into shapes. Expand your awareness and little more and the shapes come together as a painting. Expand it a little more and the painting is hanging on a wall, and the wall is in a museum, and so on. You can do this as a meditation and keep 'moving back' and expanding your awareness until your awareness isn't of the painting at all, but of the entire universe.

Now apply that same exercise to your own life. You can learn to pull back and expand your awareness of yourself and everything around you. If you've followed the exercises that I've outlined so far then you should be well on your way to making this happen.

Kundalini and Ecology

"One thing we know, which the white man may one day discover - our God is the same God. You may think now that you own Him as you wish to own our land; but you cannot. He is the God of man; and his compassion is equal for the red man and the white. This earth is precious to him and to harm the earth is to heap contempt on its Creator. The whites too shall pass; perhaps sooner than all the other tribes. Continue to contaminate your bed and you will one night suffocate in your own wastes."
From the Letter of Chief Seathl (Seattle) to the President of the United States, Franklin Pierce, 1854

Once the Kundalini begins to awaken many people suddenly develop a much closer affinity to the environment and environmental causes. The reason is quite simple. As we become more aware of our deeper connections to the world around us it makes it hard to ignore how rapidly that world is being raped and plundered by those whose only connection is to their wallet.

Working with shakti, chakras and chi is to work with the energies that surround us and that we're created from. In my case I was so attuned to those energies for a very long time that I had an extremely hard time living in the city. I had problems with this until I learned how to cleanse my energy and metabolize the *bad* energy that's so prevalent in most 'developed' areas. The realization that energy is *just energy* made this much easier.

A lot of people today are beginning to look towards Native American spirituality, Celtic and Tibetan shamanism and other paths that tend to have a closer connection to the energies and elements. There are some really good resources out there and the internet has made finding them so much easier.

Mother Earth Spirituality and *The Rainbow Tribe,* both by Ed McGaa, can be extremely helpful when you're trying to put some of your new energy into an ecological perspective.

It's hard to ignore the utter malignancy of Western Culture. It's also important to realize that many of the benefits to the modern spiritual seeker (the internet, easily available books and music, etc.) are also side effects of that culture. The challenge is to find ways to keep the benefits while creating a more sustainable lifestyle.

Us and Them

It's an interesting fact that once you begin to really open up your awareness you begin to develop a real "Us" and "Them" complex. It's important to remember that *they* are also a part of the natural order and they're even vital to our success.

Every human has the ability to awaken their Kundalini and become their true selves. It's funny that those who do are so few and far between. I think the simple fact is that even though everyone could do it, most people simply aren't meant to at this time. That's one reason I don't spend a lot of time trying to convince the skeptical about the Kundalini. I know it's real because I've experienced it firsthand. It doesn't bother me at all if others don't believe me. I'd rather put my time into empowering those who are looking for it.

The 'normal' people are just being normal and you have to love them *because* of that, rather than in spite of it. So many of the issues that plague our unenlightened society could be solved so easily through meditation and intentional living. Hopefully as the numbers of those who live intentionally increase, it'll become easier for 'them' to find the path and get onto it. The important thing to remember is that even though there are differences in perceptions of the world and life in general, there's really no such thing as 'better' or 'worse'.

Chapter 7

Epilogue: The Beginning

"Sattvic knowledge sees the one indestructible Being in all beings, the unity underlying the multiplicity of creation. Rajaistic knowledge sees all things and creatures as separate and distinct. Tamasic knowledge, lacking any sense of perspective, sees one small part and mistakes it for the whole."

-Bhagavad Gita 18:20-22
Excerpted from The Bhagavad Gita, translated by Eknath Easwaran

So where do you go from here? The answer to that is completely up to you. The journey to personal mastery is an unending saga in which we each play the starring role.

As your self-awareness grows and deepens and you become comfortable with the abilities that you develop then you may find your life going in directions that you never imagined. That's certainly been the case with me.

If you remember some of the basic principles from this book then at the very least you'll enjoy life and see it as a grand adventure, rather a than just something to survive as best you can.

In the meantime you can feel free to follow the links in the back of the book and check out the Kundalini Awakening Group I host. It's free and the whole purpose is to give people a place to ask questions and talk about their experiences.

If you liked this book then get on there and tell me so. If you didn't like it or didn't understand it then feel free to get on there and let me know that also. In later editions I'll include some questions from readers. In the meantime, have fun with your life; it's the best one you have at the moment.

Resource List for Kundalini Awakening
(These are some of the books I use on a regular basis)

Books

Pathnotes of an American Ninja Master
Dr. Glenn Morris
ISBN 1-55643-157-0

Shadow Strategies of an American Ninja Master
Dr. Glenn Morris
ISBN 1-883319-29-3

Martial Arts Madness
Dr. Glenn Morris
ISBN 1-883319-77-3

New Chakra Healing
Cyndi Dale
ISBN 1-56718-200-3

Sexual Secrets ("The Big Red Book")
Nik Douglas & Penny Slinger
ISBN 0-89281-011-4

Mother Earth Spirituality
Ed McGaa
ISBN 0-06-250596-3

The Trick to Money is Having Some
Stuart Wilde
ISBN 1-56170-168-8

Relaxing into Your Being
B.K. Frantzis
ISBN 1-55643-407-3

The Way of the Shaman
Michael Harner
ISBN 0-06-250373-1

Awaken Healing Energy Through the Tao
Mantak Chia
ISBN 0-943358-07-8

Iron Shirt Chi Kung 1
Mantak Chia
ISBN 0-935621-02-4

The Healers Manual
Ted Andrews
ISBN 0-87542-007-9

Kundalini Awakening
John Selby
ISBN 0-553-35330-6

Occult Tibet
J.M. Brennan
ISBN 0-7387-0067-3

Websites

Mystic Village Online Community
www.mysticvillage.org

The **Kundalini Awakening Discussion Group**
www.care2.com/c2c/group/Kundalini

The **Spirituality** Discussion Group
www.care2.com/c2c/group/spirituality

Mantak Chia's Universal Tao Website
www.universal-tao.com/

The *Kundalini awakening with Robert Morgen*
Podcast
www.mysticwolfpress.com

Harmony Online Magazine
www.harmonyonline.wordpress.com

Kundalini Awakening Online Magazine
www.kundaliniawakening.wordpress.com

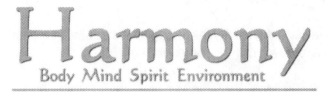

Harmony Magazine

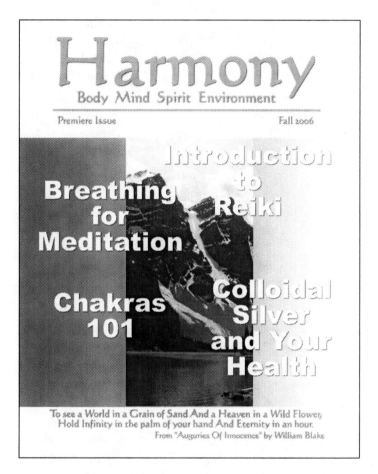

Harmony Magazine will be available in October, 2006.

Writers wanted!

We want your articles on Holistic Health, Sustainable Living, Body/Mind/Spirit, etc. Articles should be on MS Word as we also print selected articles in the new **Harmony Magazine**, the print version. Be sure to put our link on your site so people will know where to read your articles! Just link the graphic below to **http://harmonyonline.wordpress.com**

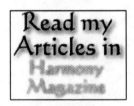

Distributors Wanted

Mystic Wolf Press needs people who are willing to take copies of Harmony Magazine to bookstores, coffee shops, yoga schools, etc. and ask for permission to leave a few copies on the counter.

We are willing to **PAY** people to do this! Payment comes in the form of free membership in the Mystic Wolf Sales Team and commissions from all of the products sold through your website, which is linked to the pages of the magazines you distribute.

For more details email Robert Morgen at:
robert@mysticwolfpress.com

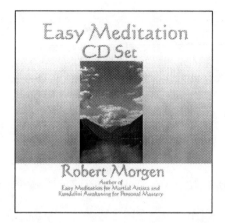

"Robert Morgen's Easy Meditation CD Set" (ISBN 0-9773801-6-5) 74.95

"Robert Morgen's Easy Meditation CD Set" is a 4 disc compilation of guided meditations and meditation exercises. Personally written and recorded by Morgen, this CD Set includes:

"Easy Introduction to Meditation"
(ISBN 0-9773801-2-2) (Running Time 66:20) $19.95

"Easy Introduction to Meditation" provides the novice through high intermediate meditator with directions, exercises and guided meditations to help one learn to clear and control the mind, develop a great degree of higher self awareness and take more control over one's life.

"Advanced Meditation Exercises"
(ISBN 0-9773801-9-X) (Running Time 74:40) $19.95

"Advanced Meditation Exercises" provides exercises and guided meditations for the high intermediate to expert meditator. Using this CD will allow one to develop stronger abilities in concentration, visualization, moving, feeling and seeing energy and much more.

"Timed Meditations"
(ISBN 0-9773801-8-1) (Running Time 76:27) $19.95

"Timed Meditations" is designed to allow one to make time for meditation in an easily controlled manner. With timed music tracks that range from 5 minutes to 25 minutes, this CD allows one to take a few minutes and meditate any time, without worrying about how much time is available.

"Opening the Chakras"
(ISBN 0-9773801-7-3) (Running Time 73:16) $29.95

"Opening the Chakras" introduces intermediate meditators to their chakra system. With brief, simple explanations Morgen guides listeners through the process of working with and opening the chakras. The powerful guided meditations on this CD have been the highlight of Morgen's Seminars and classes.

Now Available:

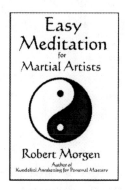

Easy Meditation for Martial Artists
By Robert Morgen

The Journey Inward

This book was created specifically for the martial artist. However, as any good martial artist can tell you, the martial arts are primarily a way to relate to and learn to live one's life at a much more intense and deeper level.

Some martial arts have very deep spiritual and meditative training already included, but in many cases the modern arts as practiced in America have had those elements removed or relegated to being practiced outside of class. It's understandable how this can happen, and I make no judgments about it.

Instead I created this book for ANY martial artist who'd like to add a deeper element to his training and life. It can be used with any style and with any technique.

The artists who incorporate these techniques into their art will find innumerable benefits to their practice and their lives in general.

Much of this book focuses on energy and how to access and use it for personal empowerment and increased abilities. Energy surrounds us. It makes up our thoughts, emotions and the physical world that we perceive. It can be measured quite easily by modern medical instruments and even seen by the naked human eye.

The ability to interact with this force, called Chi, Ki, Prana or bioelectrical energy, has been proven and documented for thousands of years.

In the martial arts we use this energy for personal development and to increase health and vitality. We also use it to access the esoteric, hidden abilities that more often than not tend to be thought of merely as myth. Learning to tap into and use this energy allows the student to be able to clear the mind, focus the intent and open up to a world that few people are even aware of.

The results can be astounding for the student who's willing to put forth the effort and delve deep into the inner worlds. While fraught with danger for the unwary and careless, the journey inward can be experienced safely and easily with a modest amount of training and a willingness to explore the inner worlds that are accessible to all.

The drills, philosophies and exercises in this book can help the serious student learn to access and use these energies. These exercises are NOT theory. In many cases the roots of the exercises are thousands of years old. They are all based on personal experience of the author and everything written about can be easily learned and experienced.

What you do with it then, is up to you.

Ask for it wherever books are sold or get it online at;

www.mysticwolfpress.com

9 780977 380107